Anesthesia for Interventional Pulmonary Procedures

Mona Sarkiss
Editor

Anesthesia for Interventional Pulmonary Procedures

Springer

Editor
Mona Sarkiss
Department of Anesthesiology and Perioperative Medicine,
Department of Pulmonary Medicine
The University of Texas MD Anderson Cancer Center
Houston, TX, USA

ISBN 978-3-032-12006-9 ISBN 978-3-032-12007-6 (eBook)
https://doi.org/10.1007/978-3-032-12007-6

This Springer imprint is published by the registered company Springer Nature Switzerland AG
The registered company address is: Gewerbestrasse 11, 6330 Cham, Switzerland

Preface

When I was asked to establish anesthesia services for interventional bronchoscopy procedures at MD Anderson Cancer Center more than two decades ago, this field was largely uncharted. I was faced with many challenges to create a safe anesthesia practice for critical airway procedures in patients with advanced airway disease away from the operating room safe environment with yet to be defined anesthesia protocols. With determination and support from my anesthesia department and Interventional Pulmonology colleagues, I pioneered one of the earliest anesthesia services for out-of-operating room bronchoscopy suites in the United States. We created an operating room replica fully equipped to deliver safe anesthesia for advanced bronchoscopic and pulmonary procedures. What began as an experiment grew into a model that is currently replicated worldwide.

I dedicated most of my anesthesia career to providing anesthesia for interventional pulmonology with the later years practicing exclusively in the bronchoscopy suite at MD Anderson Cancer Center. This book emerged to reflect my journey and experience as well as the collective wisdom of other anesthesiologists who have shaped anesthesia for Interventional Pulmonology as the subspeciality it has become today. Interventional pulmonology encompasses advanced diagnostic procedures for the diagnosis of mediastinal lymphadenopathy and lung cancer and staging of metastatic malignancies as well as therapeutic procedures for central airway obstruction and hemoptysis. Interventional pulmonary procedures are among the most complex procedures performed outside the operating room, and they require the anesthesiologists to use their technical expertise, creativity, and adaptability in a way few other settings demand.

The chapters in this book are designed to guide the reader from foundational concepts to advanced applications. The readers will find descriptions of airway strategies, anesthetic techniques, and perioperative considerations designed to complement the emerging interventional pulmonary technologies. Despite the scarcity of the available literatures, the data provided are evidence based, clinically sound, and written by experts who lived the realities of this practice.

I am deeply grateful to the authors who shared their knowledge, to the institutions and societies that continue to advance this field, and most of all to the patients whose courage inspires our work. My hope is that this volume will serve not only as a practical guide for anesthesiologists and trainees but also as an indicator of how far we have come and a foundation for the innovations yet to come.

Houston, TX, USA Mona Sarkiss

Acknowledgments

To my beloved mother, whose strength and love have guided me through every challenge.

To my devoted husband, whose unwavering support and understanding made this work possible and to my wonderful daughters, Janna and Laela—thank you for your patience and for filling my life with joy even when my long hours at work kept me away. This book is as much yours as it is mine.

I would also like to express my deepest gratitude to the Interventional Pulmonary team at MD Anderson Cancer Center, who have been my greatest teachers and collaborators throughout this journey. To Drs. Rodolfo Morice, Georgie Eapen, Carlos Jimenez, David Ost, Horiana Grosu, and Roberto Casal—thank you for sharing your expertise, your passion, and your unwavering commitment to advancing the field of interventional pulmonology. Everything I know about this specialty, I have learned from working alongside you. Your dedication and innovation continue to inspire me every day.

Contents

Introduction to Interventional Pulmonology

1

Zoulfira Nisnevitch-Savarese and Jennifer W. Toth

1.1 Introduction and Historical Perspective

Interventional pulmonology in the present represents an essential field within pulmonary medicine. These procedures encompass a wide range of diagnostic and therapeutic techniques that enable physicians to access and treat diseases of the respiratory system using minimally invasive approaches. It was not always the case. The first direct visualization of vocal cords with an autoscope was first described by Alfred Kirstein, Berlin, Germany, on April 23, 1895. Before that, the cords could be only evaluated with a small mirror, placed in patient's posterior pharynx. Kirstein had learned from his colleague that a scope intended to be passed into the esophagus had accidentally slipped into trachea and, to the surgeon's surprise, he saw a perfect view of the tracheal bifurcation. Kirstein became very interested in this finding and set to devise a method that would allow viewing larynx and trachea. He modified an esophagoscope, made it shorter, and attempted passing it following topical cocaine anesthesia of the airways. There was a problem with illumination, and he employed an electric head lamp that had been devised for examination of the urethra. However, he did not complete his development, and it was left to Gustav Killian to realize the aims of clinical use of autoscopy. In 1898, Killian performed bronchoscopy using a modified rigid oesophagoscope to remove a pig bone from the right bronchus and became regarded as the Father of Bronchoscopy [1]. The similarity between his blades and a Miller blade described in the 1940s by an anesthesiologist Robert Arden Miller is remarkable. Killian's other major contribution to laryngology was

Z. Nisnevitch-Savarese (✉)
Department of Anesthesiology, Penn State Hershey Medical Center, Hershey, PA, USA
e-mail: znisnevitchsavarese@pennstatehealth.psu.edu

J. W. Toth
Department of Medicine Division of Pulmonary, Allergy and Critical Care Medicine, Department of Surgery, Penn State Cancer Institute, Hershey, PA, USA

M. Sarkiss (ed.), *Anesthesia for Interventional Pulmonary Procedures*,
https://doi.org/10.1007/978-3-032-12007-6_1

introduction of suspension laryngoscopy. From Europe, laryngology quickly spread across the ocean, and in the same year of 1898 Algernon Coolidge from Massachusetts General Hospital was the first in America to perform a successful removal of a foreign body via bronchoscopy.

Rigid bronchoscopy as a method for direct visualization and treatment of pathological changes within the trachea and major bronchi played a key role in the advancement of thoracic surgery. During that era, thoracic surgery primarily focused on the treatment of pulmonary tuberculosis (TB). However, as the effectiveness of anti-TB medications increased, the incidence of pulmonary tuberculosis cases declined, while the prevalence of pulmonary cancer continued to rise. The rigid bronchoscope was highly valuable in identifying centrally located hilar cancers but had limited utility in diagnosing peripheral lesions below segmental branches [2].

Despite its limitations, the practice of rigid bronchoscopy remained the gold standard for seven decades until 1966 when the team led by Shigeto Ikeda, a thoracic surgeon from Tokyo, Japan, introduced the first prototype flexible fiberoptic bronchoscope. This flexible bronchoscope underwent several modifications to achieve its full functionality. The addition of a working channel, U-turn angle of 180°, addition of longer light-guide glass fiber, and an external Xenon light source rendered the sixth version of the instrument capable of accessing even the most challenging areas, including both upper lobes up to subsegmental bronchi. This was a significant advancement, given that most small cancerous lesions are typically located within the segmental and subsegmental branches of the upper lobes [2].

During that period, the flexible bronchoscope was inserted through a rigid bronchoscope or a soft endotracheal anesthesia tube. The use of the soft endotracheal tube helped minimize patient discomfort by eliminating the requirement for unnatural positioning and made prolonged examination under local anesthesia possible [2]. Bronchoscopes proved to be useful not only for the treatment of foreign body aspiration and obstructions, but also for obtaining an accurate diagnosis by tissue sampling.

Four main diagnostic tools have been developed for use during bronchoscopy to obtain diagnostic material: bronchoalveolar lavage (BAL), brushings, forceps biopsies, and needle aspirations [3].

The evolution of flexible bronchoscopes continued at a swift pace, expanding their technical capabilities and clinical utility. A notable milestone occurred in 1987 when the first flexible video bronchoscope was introduced. It featured a miniature video camera situated at the tip, enabling real-time procedure visualization on a high-definition screen and facilitating the recording of process for documentation and educational purposes [4].

The next major leap in technology happened only a few years later in the early 1990s with the introduction of endobronchial ultrasound (EBUS). An integrated fluid-filled balloon surrounding the EBUS probe created an effective interface for sound wave transmission between the ultrasound probe and the airway wall, a process known as ultrasonographic coupling. This breakthrough resolved the challenge of poor sound wave transmission in air-filled structures [3].

Endobronchial ultrasound provided the means to assess the extent of disease beyond the confines of endobronchial lesions, reaching into the pulmonary parenchyma and surrounding tissues. This resulted in an enhanced diagnostic capacity for pulmonary masses, nodules, and intrathoracic adenopathy, diminishing the necessity for more invasive surgical interventions.

Further significant technological advances led to the development of a wide array of diverse modern interventional procedures that will be reviewed next.

1.2 Techniques and Procedures

1.2.1 Flexible Bronchoscopy

Bronchoalveolar lavage (BAL), bronchial brushings, transbronchial biopsy (TBB), and transbronchial needle aspiration (TBNA) are the basic diagnostic procedures conducted during fiberoptic bronchoscopy.

When performing a BAL, the bronchoscope is gently wedged into the target bronchus, while maintaining the view of the lumen of the bronchus. Aliquots of 30–60 mL of sterile normal saline are instilled into the alveoli for a total of at least 100 mL and a maximum of 240 mL. Subsequently, the fluid is aspirated into a collection trap, with pressure maintained below 100 mmHg adjusted to prevent visible airway collapse.

In a healthy nonsmoking individual, the cellular composition of BAL typically includes macrophages (80–90%), lymphocytes (5–15%) with a CD4/CD8 ratio ranging from 1.5 to 1.8, neutrophils (1–3%), and eosinophils and mast cells at levels below 1% [5]. BAL plays an important role in the diagnosis of pulmonary infections, particularly in immunocompromised individuals and cases of mycobacterial infections [6].

A combination of BAL with transbronchial biopsy and bronchial brushings increases the diagnostic yield for microbiological and cytological samples of small peripheral lung nodules measuring less than 2 cm. The brushings involve the insertion of a small brush via the flexible bronchoscope directed toward a visible endoluminal lesion or a peripheral pulmonary nodule with the aid of fluoroscopy, radial EBUS, or virtual bronchoscopy techniques [7].

Transbronchial lung biopsy (TBLB) refers to sampling the lung parenchyma using flexible biopsy forceps. TBLB and lung cryobiopsy are valuable tools in the evaluation of interstitial lung disease (ILD), aiding in accurate diagnosis and guiding treatment decisions. Typically, this procedure begins by wedging the bronchoscope into the bronchus. The biopsy forceps are then carefully advanced in a closed position through the bronchoscope's working channel, guided by fluoroscopy, until resistance is encountered. The forceps are gently pulled back approximately 1 cm, opened, and then readvanced until the desired tissue is in contact with the forceps, at which point they are closed again to obtain a biopsy sample.

TBLB is associated with a low rate of complications, including major bleeding (greater than 50 mL) in less than 1% of cases and a risk of pneumothorax ranging between 1% and 4% [8–10].

Blind transbronchial needle aspiration (TBNA) involves the collection of samples through the tracheal or bronchial wall and can be utilized to sample mediastinal and hilar lymph nodes as well as lung and mediastinal masses. It is performed under fluoroscopy guidance. Before proceeding with this method, it is crucial to conduct a comprehensive review of the patient's chest computed tomography (CT) and possess a sound understanding of thoracic anatomy. A retractable hollow cytology needle (21 or 22 gauge) or histology needle (19 gauge) is employed, with suction applied at the proximal end. The sensitivity of blind TBNA can vary based on factors such as the size and location of the lesion, the number of aspirates per lymph node, and the operator's level of experience. Notably, the overall complication rate for blind TBNA remains quite low at 0.8% [11]. The introduction of EBUS-TBNA for mediastinal and hilar adenopathy and central tumors has significantly reduced the reliance on blind TBNA.

An analysis of 30 studies, published in 2003, aimed to evaluate the performance characteristics of various diagnostic methods for suspected lung cancer. The combined diagnostic yield of all these methods for central endobronchial disease was found to be 88%. Among these methods, endobronchial biopsy exhibited the highest sensitivity at 74% [12].

In cases of peripheral lung lesions, cytobrush displayed the highest sensitivity at 52%, followed by transbronchial biopsy at 46%, and BAL/washings at 43%. The overall sensitivity for all the diagnostic methods was 69%. Notably, when considering peripheral lesions with diameters less than 2 cm, the sensitivities were poor (33%) [12].

1.2.2 Endobronchial Ultrasound

Endobronchial ultrasound utilizes an integrated fluid-filled latex balloon that envelops the EBUS probe, creating a medium interface capable of transmitting sound waves for ultrasound imaging (termed ultrasonographic coupling). The ultrasound frequency is important for EBUS applications. Lower frequencies offer enhanced penetration depth but lower resolution, while higher frequencies provide superior spatial resolution but reduced penetration depth. In EBUS applications, the frequency range typically falls between 7.5 and 30 MHz. There are currently three types of EBUS probes available, each designed for specific applications: (1) convex probe or curvilinear EBUS (CP EBUS), (2) radial balloon probe (20 MHz), and (3) ultra-miniature radial probes (20 and 30 MHz).

The convex probe bronchoscope has a larger distal diameter (6.9 mm) compared to standard therapeutic bronchoscopes (6.2 mm) (Fig. 1.1) and is equipped with an integrated ultrasound probe that scans perpendicular to the longitudinal axis, offering a 90° US view. It also provides a forward oblique video view of 35° and a 2.0-mm working channel, facilitating the passage of a dedicated biopsy needle (21- or 22-gauge). The biopsy needle used with this probe is designed with distal indentations that reflect ultrasound waves, enhancing needle visualization (Figs. 1.2 and 1.3).

The radial balloon EBUS (Fig. 1.4) offers remarkable resolution of less than 1 mm and provides a 360° visualization of paratracheal and peribronchial

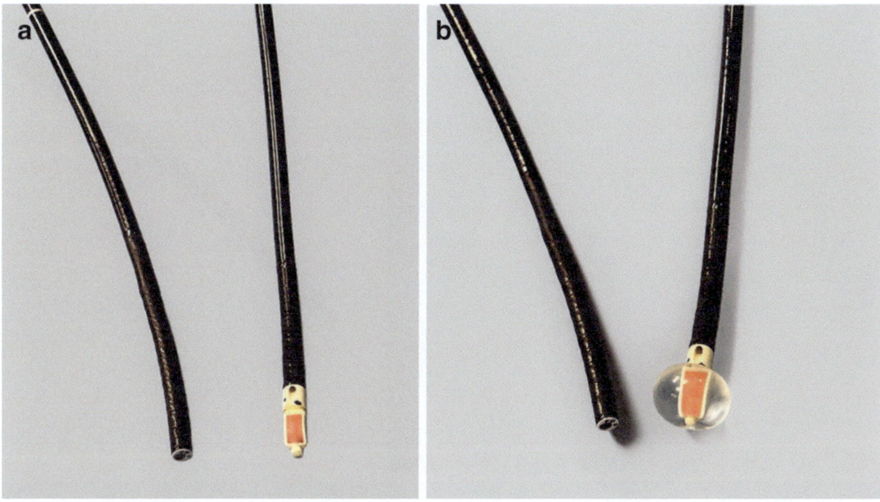

Fig. 1.1 (**a**) Therapeutic bronchoscope (left) compared to convex probe bronchoscope (right). (**b**) Therapeutic bronchoscope (left) compared to endobronchial ultrasound probe with balloon inflated (right)

Fig. 1.2 Endobronchial ultrasound probe with a biopsy needle

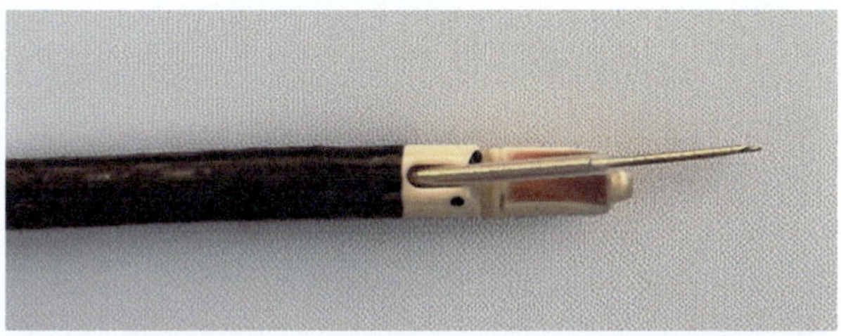

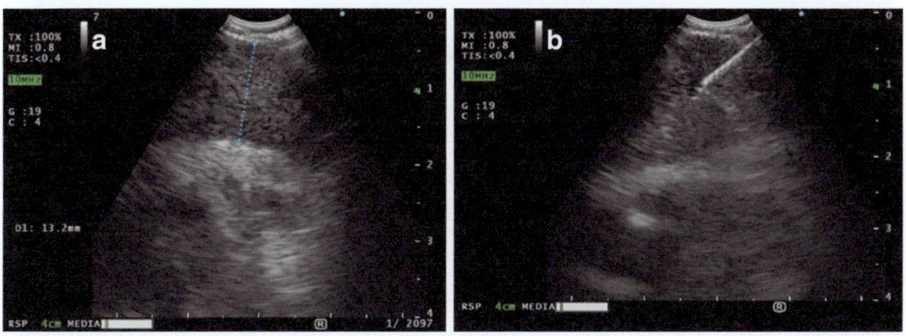

Fig. 1.3 (**a**) Endobronchial ultrasound image of mediastinal mass. (**b**) Endobronchial ultrasound image of a needle in a mediastinal mass

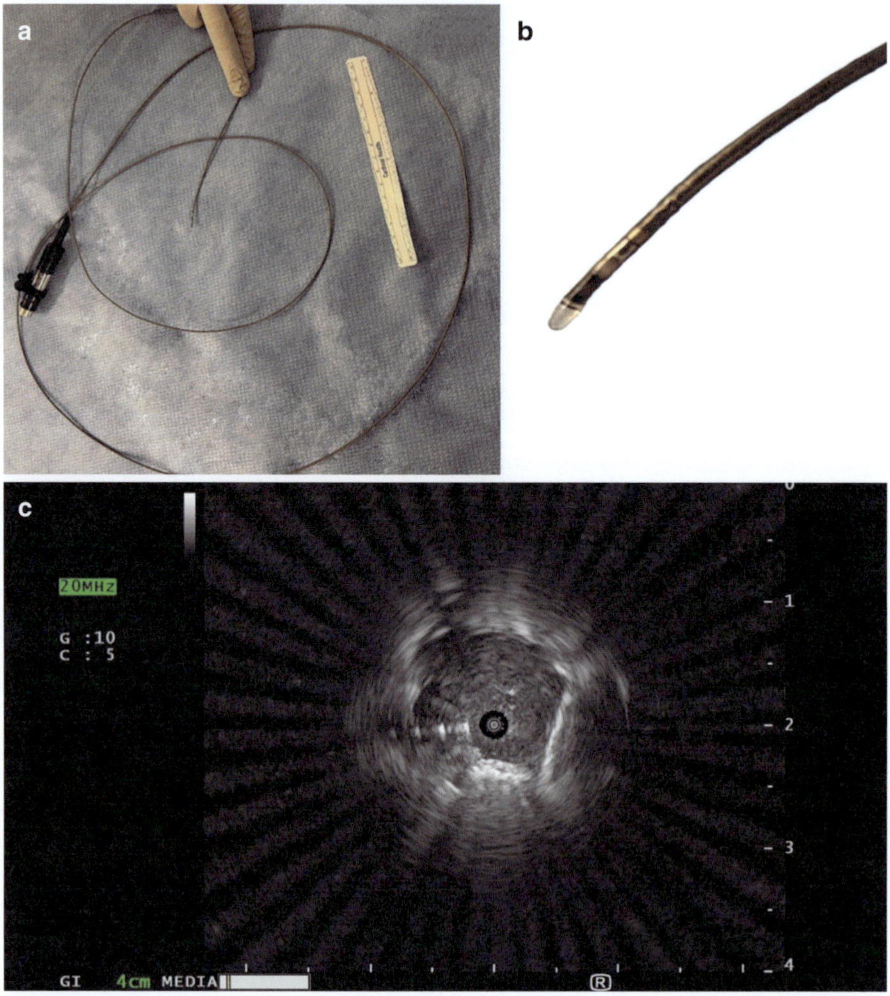

Fig. 1.4 (**a**, **b**) Radial probe. (**c**) Ultrasonic view of a mass captured by a radial probe

structures. The RB-EBUS demonstrates a high sensitivity (93–95%) in determining airway wall involvement in cases of malignancy [13, 14]. It significantly outperforms CT scans in differentiating airway involvement, improving diagnostic accuracy from 51% to 94% [15]. This superior performance has also been observed in patients with thyroid or esophageal cancer, where tracheal involvement was a concern [16]. These studies highlight the RB-EBUS's capacity to stage tumors in a minimally invasive manner, surpassing the capabilities of other imaging modalities and thereby reducing the need for exploratory thoracotomies [3].

The ultra-miniature (UM)-EBUS contains a circulating ultrasound crystal that provides a 360° view of the surrounding structures when full airway ultrasonographic coupling is established. The compact size and extensive field of view allow the UM-EBUS to dramatically improve sensitivity for small parenchymal lesions [3, 17]. This probe is inserted through a sheath, which can remain in the airway upon UM-EBUS probe removal to guide instruments for a more successful biopsy.

1.2.3 Navigational Techniques

Other navigational techniques have recently emerged to address the challenge of bronchoscopic localization for small peripheral pulmonary lesions, which were previously only accessible through CT-guided transthoracic needle biopsy (TTNB). While TTNB boasts a diagnostic accuracy ranging from 84% to 97%, it carries a significant risk of complications, such as pneumothorax (15–30%), and subjects patients to considerable discomfort. Various modalities of navigational bronchoscopy have been developed. The first FDA-approved system is based on electromagnetic navigation (EMN) (e.g., InReach System from SuperDimension, Ltd.). It utilizes an electromagnetic board to create a magnetic field around the patient, a position sensor probe, an extended working channel, and real-time three-dimensional reconstructions of previously acquired CT images with the position of the bronchoscope. This EMN system operates based on the triangulation principle similar to a global positioning system (GPS) and guides the bronchoscopist through the airways to the target. Several studies have shown that EMN offers diagnostic sensitivity ranging from 67% to 74%, independent of lesion size and location [18, 19]. EMN accuracy is subject to electromagnetic interference from metal objects in the operating room.

Combining navigational bronchoscopy with endobronchial ultrasound and cone-beam CT (CBCT) allows for simultaneous EBUS nodal staging, enhances physicians' ability to reach peripheral lung lesions, and facilitates more precise tissue sampling [20]. In contrast to conventional spiral CT imaging, which uses a fan-shaped X-ray beam and multiple linear detectors taking multiple images, while a patient is moved through the machine, CBCT employs a cone-shaped X-ray and a single area detector capable of capturing a full volume of image in a single rotation, eliminating the need to move the patient. CBCT can be quickly performed with a C-Arm, and its single-image capture reduces radiation exposure to both the patient and staff [21].

Robotic-assisted bronchoscopy (RAB) represents an attempt to further address and improve upon the challenges encountered during conventional and EMN procedures.

1.2.4 Robotic-Assisted Bronchoscopy

Two FDA-approved robotic-assisted bronchoscopy platforms currently available are the Monarch by Auris Health, using electromagnetic (EM) guidance, and the Ion Robotic Endoluminal platform by Intuitive Surgical, employing Shape Sensing Technology. Both platforms have a robotic cart with arms for holding a flexible bronchoscope and electronic systems with monitors capable of generating 3D maps and providing real-time precise location fused with preoperative CT imaging. Intraoperative fluoroscopy and radial EBUS are frequently utilized together with RAB to improve diagnostic yield [22].

The Monarch platform combines three distinct navigation technologies—electromagnetics, optical pattern recognition, and robotic kinematic data—to navigate a catheter to the nodule via a pathway directed by a preprocedural CT [23]. The 4.2 mm OD bronchoscope is similar in size to conventional thin bronchoscopes but can articulate up to 180° in any direction, allowing access to the most distant areas. It is advanced through a 6 mm outer sheath that can also be articulated up to 130° and is held by the robotic arms. Physician maneuvers the scope with the help of a videogame-type controller. The configuration has a 2.1 mm working channel for various instruments. Real-time video captured from the bronchoscope's tip is overlaid with CT imaging and other information from the robotic system and is displayed on the tower monitor. The electromagnetic field generator placed close to the patient's chest, together with reference sensors attached to the patient's chest, allows triangulation of the location of a scope relative to the target lesion. The largest multicenter study with the Monarch platform included 167 lesions with a successful navigation rate of 88.6% and a diagnostic yield of 69–77%. Bleeding was reported in 2.4% of cases and a pneumothorax rate of 3.6% [23, 24].

The Ion Endoluminal System uses shape-sensing technology and does not rely on electromagnetic navigation; hence, it is not subject to interference from nearby metal objects. The flexible bronchoscope is smaller, with an outer diameter 3.5 mm and a working channel of 2.0 mm. The removable vision probe is placed within the catheter. The robotic catheter also articulates 180° in all directions. Shape-sensing fibers within the scope give positional feedback on precise location and distance to the target. The robot cart has display screens that can project bronchoscopic and radial ultrasound views. Finally, there is a controller cart with a trackball and scroll wheel. Robotic bronchoscopy is frequently combined with cone-beam CT and r-EBUS to further improve the diagnostic yield.

EMN and RAB applications can also be used for the delivery of targeted cancer therapeutic agents, implantation of radiotherapy monitoring devices, and lesion dye marking or stereotactic radiosurgery fiducial placement to guide surgical resections [25].

1.2.5 Pleuroscopy/Medical Thoracoscopy

The method of "examination of interior of pleura by endoscope" was documented as early as 1866. Francis-Richard Cruise, hailing from Dublin, Ireland, is believed to be likely the first to perform a thoracoscopy through a pleurocutaneous fistula in an 11-year-old girl with empyema. He utilized this technique to monitor progress of the therapy. Although it was published in the *Dublin Quarterly Journal of Medical Science*, the technique remained anecdotal until 1910 when Hans-Christian Jacobaeus developed and described thoracoscopy as a diagnostic method [26]. The term "medical thoracoscopy" was introduced in 1994 by Mathur et al. This term is commonly used to describe procedures utilizing small rigid instruments for the examination of the pleural cavity. Conversely, the term "pleuroscopy" suggests the use of flexible scopes and instruments to visualize the pleural cavity, conduct biopsies, perform nonsurgical pleurodesis, and manage other pleural diseases [26].

Given its more invasive nature, this procedure should be reserved to obtain diagnosis when other less invasive methods have proven nondiagnostic. It does not require tracheal intubation and lung isolation and can be performed under local anesthesia or sedation.

1.2.6 Therapeutic Procedures via Fiberoptic Bronchoscopy

Several groundbreaking tools, methods, and revolutionary designs are available for therapeutic procedures using fiberoptic bronchoscopy. Their application enables interventions for previously fatal conditions, enhancing patient life expectancy and decreasing the necessity for high-risk airway surgeries.

1.2.6.1 Laser Therapy

Used to treat airway tumors and strictures, laser therapy involves the precise destruction of abnormal tissue using laser energy. The first clinical application of laser in the respiratory tract was reported in 1973 with the carbon dioxide (CO2) laser [27]. Since then, several lasers such as argon and KTP have also been used. In 1981, Dumon described use of endobronchial Nd-YAG laser [28, 29]. It remains the most commonly utilized laser type for endobronchial tumors. Nd-YAG is preferred for its deeper tissue penetration, sufficient energy range to vaporize lesions at high power while producing coagulation at low power. Its wavelength is less absorbed by hemoglobin and quartz. The latter feature allows it to be transmitted by a flexible fiber [30]. The laser fiber is introduced through the working channel of the FB. The laser fiber tip should be at least 4 mm away from both the target lesion and the distal end of the bronchoscope. The inspired FiO2 should be lowered to 40% or less to minimize the risk of endobronchial fire, and frequent suctioning should be used to remove the combustible laser plume [30]. Laser therapy can be performed via either rigid or flexible bronchoscopy. The flexible bronchoscope is useful to treat smaller lesions. Severe obstruction or critical situations are better handled with the rigid bronchoscope. Complications related to laser application include hemorrhage (1.6–3%), pneumothorax (0.1–0.3%), endobronchial fire (0.1–0.2%), and periprocedural death (1–2%) [31].

1.2.6.2 Electrocautery (FBE)

Electrocautery is another modality to treat central airway obstructions from benign or malignant tumors of the airway. It also acts through coagulation and vaporization and can be used as a probe and as a snare. The electrical probe is used to treat superficial lesions, while the snare is applied to polypoid tumors in the airway lumen. Data suggest that FBE is equally effective as Nd:YAG laser and is a cheaper and simpler tool for obtaining tumor clearance [32]. Complications are like those of laser application, with bleeding being the most common [32, 33]. Suggested settings to avoid fire during the procedure are FiO2 equal to or less than 40% and low power (20–30 W).

1.2.6.3 Argon Plasma Coagulation (APC)

APC is a noncontact electrocautery that uses ionized argon to transmit high-frequency electrical current to cause coagulation and vaporization. It has less penetration compared with Nd:YAG laser. It has been used in surgery for more than 30 years, particularly for the hemostasis of superficial bleeding. It is commonly used to treat bleeding exophytic endobronchial tumors with a reported success rate of 99% in managing hemoptysis [34]. APC can also be applied to other benign lesions compromising the airway, such as granulomas resulting from airway stents, and has been successfully applied to recanalize occluded stents. It is commonly used in conjunction with other techniques.

Reported complications related to APC are hemorrhage, airway perforation, gas embolism, and airway fire [35].

1.2.6.4 Cryobiopsy/Cryotherapy

This technique involves freezing and extracting samples of diseased tissues within the airways. Cryosurgical equipment functions based on the Joule–Thomson effect, where, if a highly compressed gas in a liquid state is released at a high flow rate, it undergoes rapid expansion, resulting in an extremely low temperature. The most commonly used cryogenic agents are carbon dioxide (CO2) or nitrous oxide. The gas at the tip expands due to the sudden difference in pressure relative to the atmospheric pressure, resulting in a drop of temperature at the tip of the probe (around −80 °C). The size of cryobiopsies correlates positively with longer activation time and larger size of the cryoprobe that comes at a diameter of 1.1, 1.7, 1.9, or 2.4 mm.

Cryotherapy can also be used as a therapeutic intervention to treat obstruction or growth in airways, mostly for palliation. In these cases, cycles of freezing and thawing are applied to the target, causing delayed necrosis. Cryotherapy does not open airway rapidly and is not commonly used in critical airway obstruction since generated edema may worsen the degree of obstruction [36].

Transbronchial lung cryobiopsy to diagnose and guide treatment of interstitial lung disease is performed in some institutions, where cryoprobe is introduced into the selected lung area under fluoroscopic guidance via a flexible or rigid bronchoscope. A distance of approximately 10–20 mm from the thoracic wall is considered optimal. Once the probe's tip is at the target area, the probe is activated for approximately 3–6 s. The frozen tissue attached to the probe's tip is removed by pulling the bronchoscope and cryoprobe together. It is important to recognize the higher rate of potential complications, such as pneumothorax and bleeding when using TBLC. Placing a bronchial blocker before the cryobiopsy and inflating it immediately after the probe is removed had helped decrease the risk of significant hemorrhage. Therefore, TBLC/cryotherapy should be performed by interventional pulmonologists who are trained to manage potential complications.

1.2.6.5 Airway Stenting

Stents are indicated for intraluminal obstruction, stenosis, extrinsic compression, expiratory central airway collapse or tracheomalacia, bronchial fistula, or dehiscence. Both rigid and flexible bronchoscopy can be utilized to place airway stents. The flexible bronchoscope can be used to deploy self-expandable metallic stents (SEMS) in the airway. Both bare and fully covered SEMS are commercially available.

The bare SEMS are more commonly used for malignant conditions. Long-term presence of a stent inside the airway has been linked to severe complications such as erosion and perforation of the airway wall, excessive granulation tissue, bacterial colonization, stent disruption, and fracture [37, 38]. Bronchial dehiscence and post-surgical stenosis following lung transplant or tracheal resection are a few indications for the deployment of metallic stents to promote granulation tissue formation and healing. In those cases, the stents are exchanged every 2–3 weeks to prevent stent integration into airway.

Silicone stents are recommended for benign obstructions for their ease of repositioning and removal, with the major drawbacks being stent migration, stent obstruction, reduction in airway diameter due to thick stent wall, and a need for rigid bronchoscopy for placement and removal [39, 40].

The Food and Drug Administration (FDA) released recommendations regarding the use of metallic airway stents for benign disease in 2005. Experts recommend avoiding bare metallic stents for benign disease and considering other therapeutic strategies [37] such as balloon dilation.

1.2.6.6 Bronchoscopic Lung Volume Reduction

A minimally invasive procedure aimed at reducing hyperinflation and improving quality of life in certain patients with severe emphysema, who are refractory to conventional treatment. The technique involves the insertion of endobronchial valves, or historically, coils, into designated airways to block nonfunctional segments, thus improving V/Q matching and allowing more efficient ventilation of healthier portions of the lung. Another indication for valve placement is a nonsurgical treatment of persistent air leaks.

Valves are the most effective in patients with complete fissure and absence of collateral ventilation to the target lobe [41].

Two FDA-approved endobronchial one-way valves are commercially available:

Zephyr valve: A silicone duckbill-shaped valve attached to Nitinol self-expandable frame (Fig. 1.5).

Spiration valve: An umbrella-shaped self-expanding valve made of various metals, including a nickel–titanium frame. Distal anchors secure the valve against bronchial walls, with proximal struts keeping contact with the airway.

The valves come in various sizes to fit target airway size. They can be passed through a flexible bronchoscope with a channel larger than 2.6 mm.

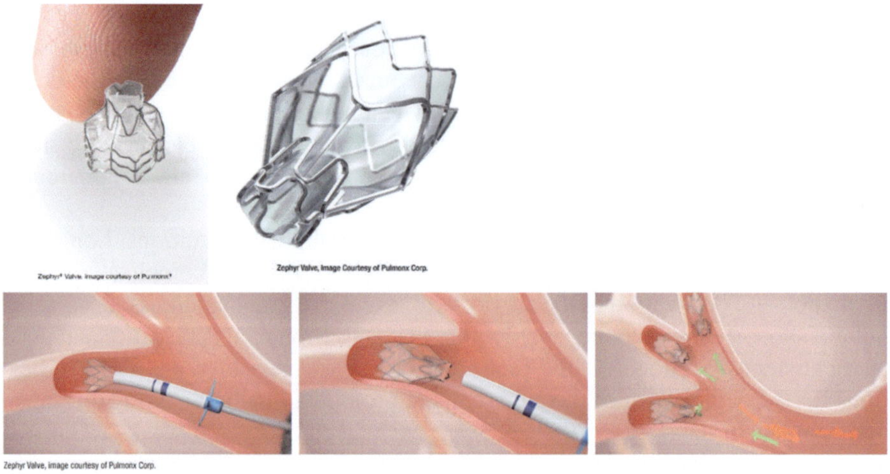

Fig. 1.5 Zephyr valve. (Image courtesy of Pulmonix Corp)

1.3 Evolution of Anesthesia Techniques for Pulmonary Interventions

The main advancement in anesthesiology started with the development of tools for airway management. In that respect, anesthesia and interventional pulmonology have the same founding fathers. Alfred Kirstein, Gustav Killian, and Chevalier Jackson paved the way to modern airway management.

Pennsylvania-born Chevalier Jackson devised a lighted bronchoscope and several instruments for foreign body removal. He was a professor at six different schools, including the University of Pittsburgh, Jefferson Medical College, Women's Medical College (now Drexel University College of Medicine), and Temple University.

Jackson was the first to describe the combination of direct visualization of the larynx with his handheld laryngoscope and the passage of an endotracheal tube with a high rate of success, and its popularity quickly caught hold after 1913.

Despite the introduction of ether by William T.G. Morton on October 16, 1846, and nitrous oxide mixed with oxygen by Edmund Andrews in 1856, rigid laryngoscopy and bronchoscopy were performed under local anesthesia with cocaine even in the early 1900s. Cocaine produced many side effects and was considered "poisonous" by many. The optimal anesthetics for patient comfort were lacking at that time, which restricted general application of this valuable technique. Between 1900 and the 1940s, most of the surgical procedures were performed with local or regional anesthesia. The only available local anesthetic besides cocaine was procaine. It had a short duration of action and high incidence of toxic effects. Lidocaine was invented in the 1940s at the Karolinska Institute in Stockholm and was overwhelmingly superior to any available local anesthetics. It became the most used local anesthetic for bronchoscopy due to its duration of action and safety profile.

With the invention of barbiturates as an intravenous anesthetic in 1932, general anesthesia started to be used for interventional bronchoscopy, markedly improving patient safety and satisfaction. Use of general anesthesia with LMA or tracheal intubation and mechanical ventilation allowed more complex and precise bronchoscopic procedures to be performed safely and more comfortably for the patients and the proceduralists.

1.4 Role of Anesthesia in Interventional Pulmonology

As bronchoscopy has traditionally been conducted under topical anesthesia, a significant shift in mindset and the accumulation of evidence were necessary to introduce sedation and general anesthesia into the field. The debate over whether to use sedation or not started in the early 1990s.

A retrospective study, published in 1990, evaluated the safety of FOB with and without premedication regimen. Of the 281 bronchoscopies, 91 were performed without premedication, while 191 were conducted with premedication, a choice even acknowledged by the authors as a selection bias. The premedication regimen was based on physician preferences and consisted of either intramuscularly administered codeine and atropine; meperidine, hydroxyzine, and atropine; or intramuscularly administered atropine and intravenously administered diazepam. The study recommended that routine diagnostic FOB (excluding transbronchial biopsy) be performed without premedication. This approach was advocated to decrease facility fees, reduce medication and personnel costs, and diminish the need for postprocedure observation, all without compromising patient care, safety, or comfort [42].

In another prospective randomized double-blind study dated 1994, three patient groups undergoing diagnostic FOB without transbronchial biopsy were compared. The findings revealed no significant differences in benefits among patients who received phenoperidine and droperidol, those who received midazolam titrated for light sedation, and those given a placebo [43].

These results fueled the notion that sedation was an avoidable factor that could contribute to additional costs and potentially compromise patient safety.

With the development of new intravenous anesthetics with shorter duration of effect and improved pharmacological profiles, it became evident that the addition of conscious sedation offered a significant reduction in discomfort and an improvement in patient satisfaction, while carrying a slight but manageable risk of hypoxemia during FOB [44, 45]. As a result, the utilization of sedation during these procedures increased from 51% in 1991 to 73% in 2003 [46]. Additional research has shown that, in addition to improved satisfaction, sedated patients experienced a decrease in cough and laryngospasm [47]. Typically, anesthesia providers are not directly involved in these procedures and sedation is administered by proceduralists, nurses, respiratory therapists, and others [48, 49].

In 2011, the American College of Chest Physicians released a Consensus Statement on the Use of Topical Anesthesia, Analgesia, and Sedation During Flexible Bronchoscopy in Adult Patients, concluding that "there is an equal safety record of sedation vs no sedation in bronchoscopy, but patients' satisfaction and procedure tolerance are significantly improved with sedation" and suggesting sedation to be used in all patients undergoing bronchoscopy unless contraindications exist.

According to a self-reported survey from 2016 in Switzerland, propofol was the most commonly used agent. For 84% of respondents, propofol was administered without an anesthesiologist present. While monitoring vital parameters has become standard practice, pulmonologists reported a very low rate of systematic basic education and training in the field of PSA (50%). Of those physicians who used propofol, 43% reported that they were actively supported or trained by an anesthesiologist at the time of the introduction of the drug [49]. Practices vary widely between countries and even between different facilities in the same country.

More complex bronchoscopic procedures involving biopsies and other instrumentation demand a high degree of precision and the imperative need to prevent coughing and patient movement. As a result, these procedures are typically conducted under general anesthesia in a specialized facility or setting.

There is a clear benefit of having expert anesthesia team performing anesthesia and sedation in the interventional pulmonology suite. Licensed anesthesia providers are adept at creating the best conditions for a procedure to be successful. By maintaining patient safety and comfort, they allow the interventionalist to concentrate entirely on the procedure. With a dramatic increase in the variety and complexity of bronchoscopic procedures, the familiarity of anesthesia providers with every aspect of the procedure becomes increasingly crucial. Close communication between teams, ability to anticipate the next steps or potential complications, and readiness to promptly treat them are paramount.

One of the distinctive challenges in interventional pulmonology arises from the shared airway during bronchoscopy. This dynamic implies an interprofessional team working closely in a limited space, where the anesthesiologist may not always have immediate access to the patient. Furthermore, the use of jet ventilation, especially during rigid bronchoscopy, has become more common. Jet ventilation through a rigid bronchoscope necessitates constant vigilance and places less reliance on monitors since it does not allow precise measuring of delivered ventilation. Instead, anesthesia providers must rely on vital signs and visual assessment to ensure effective ventilation, making their role even more critical.

The wide array of modern tools and medications offers extensive options for anesthesia administration. The choices depend on patient factors, provider preference, proceduralist goals and preference, level of expertise, environmental considerations, and various other factors. High-flow nasal cannula (HFNC) with total intravenous anesthesia can be utilized for a simple bronchoscopy in patients with stable baseline oxygenation; however, in patients with respiratory failure, HFNC was shown to be inferior to noninvasive ventilation [50].

The airway can be supported using a supraglottic airway (SGA) or an endotracheal tube (ETT). A laryngeal mask airway is a widely employed option as it enables adequate examination of the larynx and facilitates sampling of high-level (e.g., station 2) mediastinal lymph nodes. LMA is also preferred to endotracheal intubation in patients with tracheal stenosis or tumors, in whom an endotracheal tube placement can be difficult and traumatic [51]. The LMA for bronchoscopy should have a short round lumen, big enough to fit a 6.9 mm external diameter bronchoscope while allowing adequate ventilation. Presence of a built-in bite block to prevent inadvertent biting and damage to equipment is also important. The presence of an esophageal port helps decrease the risk of aspiration and stomach distention. Other SGAs (e.g., i-gel®) have also been successfully used [52]. Furthermore, the LMA offers the advantage of allowing for the passage of an ETT in case of emergency.

The LMA Supreme has an oval-shaped lumen that cannot accommodate the passage of a bronchoscope; therefore, its use should be avoided.

Endotracheal intubation with positive pressure ventilation might be beneficial or even necessary in cases where the patient's airway precludes proper LMA placement or when the passage of tools through vocal cords (VC) has the potential of VC damage, such as the insertion endobronchial valves [53] or stents. In the latter case, the ETT should be positioned under direct vision and secured above the level of intervention to facilitate access without interfering with stent deployment. The internal diameter of the ETT should exceed 8.0 mm to accommodate a large bronchoscope without compromising ventilation.

Rigid bronchoscopy requires unique approaches to ventilation, such as apneic ventilation, manual, or high-frequency jet ventilation.

Pharmacological approaches vary based on the indication for bronchoscopy and the complexity of the case. Commonly employed combinations include but are not limited to propofol + remifentanil; propofol + other opioid (fentanyl/alfentanil); midazolam+ fentanyl; propofol +rocuronium [52, 54]. Use of topical lidocaine is recommended with all these combinations. Addition of ketamine or dexmedetomidine has been described with a variable degree of success [46, 54–57]. The use of muscle relaxants presents advantages, such as the prevention of laryngospasm and the facilitation of bronchoscopy by maintaining the vocal cords in the adducted position. Additionally, muscle paralysis eliminates the risk of coughing and patient movements during the procedure [58]. This can also help prevent hemodynamic instability by reducing the need for intraoperative opioids. However, it is important to note that intact inspiratory muscle tone plays a vital role in maintaining alveolar expansion, so the use of muscle relaxants may pose a higher risk of atelectasis [59]. When relaxants are used, adequate and prompt reversal at the conclusion of the procedure must be assured.

Use of inhalational anesthesia is discouraged since frequent suctioning, manipulation of bronchoscopes, and circuit leakage can lead to unreliable drug delivery, intraoperative recall, and contamination of the operative room [58]. For these reasons, use of bispectral index (BIS) monitor is encouraged to monitor the depth of anesthesia irrespective of the type of anesthetic [60, 61]. Despite its equivocal reliability [62], monitoring BIS or EEG can guide titration of anesthetics to minimize overdosing and hemodynamic instability.

1.5 Conclusion

Interventional pulmonary procedures have transformed the diagnosis and management of various respiratory disorders. By combining innovation with minimally invasive approaches, these procedures offer patients less invasive options, quicker recovery times, and improved outcomes. As technology continues to advance, the field of interventional pulmonary procedures will undoubtedly expand, further enhancing our ability to diagnose and treat respiratory diseases. In the subsequent chapters of this book, we will delve deeper into specific procedures, their techniques, complications, and evolving trends in this exciting and dynamic field.

References

1. Becker H. History of the rigid bronchoscope. In: Bolliger CT, Mathur PN, editors. Interventional bronchoscopy. Basel: Karger; 2000. p. 2–15.
2. Ikeda S, Yanai N, Ishikawa S. Flexible bronchofiberscope. Keio J Med. 1968;1(17):1–16.
3. Haas AR, Vachani A, Sterman DH. Advances in diagnostic bronchoscopy. Am J Respir Crit Care Med. 2010;182(5):589–97. https://doi.org/10.1164/rccm.201002-0186CI.
4. Miyazawa T, Miyazu Y, Iwamoto Y. Interventional flexible bronchoscopy. Historical perspective. In: Beamis J, Mathur P, A M, editors. Interventional pulmonary medicine lung biology in health and disease. New York: Marcel Dekker; 2004. p. 33–48.
5. Heron M, Grutters JC, ten Dam-Molenkamp KM, et al. Bronchoalveolar lavage cell pattern from healthy human lung. Clin Exp Immunol. 2012;167(3):523–31. https://doi.org/10.1111/j.1365-2249.2011.04529.x.
6. Joos L, Chhajed PN, Wallner J, et al. Pulmonary infections diagnosed by BAL: a 12-year experience in 1066 immunocompromised patients. Respir Med. 2007;101(1):93–7. https://doi.org/10.1016/j.rmed.2006.04.006.
7. Boonsarngsuk V, Kanoksil W, Laungdamerongchai S. Comparison of diagnostic performances among bronchoscopic sampling techniques in the diagnosis of peripheral pulmonary lesions. J Thorac Dis. 2015;7(4):697–703. https://doi.org/10.3978/j.issn.2072-1439.2015.04.31.
8. Pajares V, Núñez-Delgado M, Bonet G, et al. Transbronchial biopsy results according to diffuse interstitial lung disease classification. Cryobiopsy versus forceps: MULTICRIO study. PLoS One. 2020;15(9):e0239114. https://doi.org/10.1371/journal.pone.0239114.
9. Tukey MH, Wiener RS. Population-based estimates of transbronchial lung biopsy utilization and complications. Respir Med. 2012;106(11):1559–65. https://doi.org/10.1016/j.rmed.2012.08.008.
10. Ito T, Okachi S, Iwano S, et al. Diagnostic value and safety of endobronchial ultrasonography with a guide sheath transbronchial biopsy for diagnosing peripheral pulmonary lesions in patients with interstitial lung disease. J Thorac Dis. 2022;14(11):4361–71. https://doi.org/10.21037/jtd-22-809.
11. Holty JE, Kuschner WG, Gould MK. Accuracy of transbronchial needle aspiration for mediastinal staging of non-small cell lung cancer: a meta-analysis. Thorax. 2005;60(11):949–55. https://doi.org/10.1136/thx.2005.041525.

12. Schreiber G, McCrory DC. Performance characteristics of different modalities for diagnosis of suspected lung cancer: summary of published evidence. Chest. 2003;123(1 Suppl):115S–28S. https://doi.org/10.1378/chest.123.1_suppl.115s.
13. Kurimoto N, Murayama M, Yoshioka S, et al. Assessment of usefulness of endobronchial ultrasonography in determination of depth of tracheobronchial tumor invasion. Chest. 1999;115(6):1500–6. https://doi.org/10.1378/chest.115.6.1500.
14. Tanaka F, Muro K, Yamasaki S, et al. Evaluation of tracheo-bronchial wall invasion using transbronchial ultrasonography (TBUS). Eur J Cardiothorac Surg. 2000;17(5):570–4. https://doi.org/10.1016/s1010-7940(00)00372-9.
15. Herth F, Ernst A, Schulz M, et al. Endobronchial ultrasound reliably differentiates between airway infiltration and compression by tumor. Chest. 2003;123(2):458–62. https://doi.org/10.1378/chest.123.2.458.
16. Wakamatsu T, Tsushima K, Yasuo M, et al. Usefulness of preoperative endobronchial ultrasound for airway invasion around the trachea: esophageal cancer and thyroid cancer. Respiration. 2006;73(5):651–7. https://doi.org/10.1159/000093160.
17. Yamada N, Yamazaki K, Kurimoto N, et al. Factors related to diagnostic yield of transbronchial biopsy using endobronchial ultrasonography with a guide sheath in small peripheral pulmonary lesions. Chest. 2007;132(2):603–8. https://doi.org/10.1378/chest.07-0637.
18. Gildea TR, Mazzone PJ, Karnak D, et al. Electromagnetic navigation diagnostic bronchoscopy: a prospective study. Am J Respir Crit Care Med. 2006;174(9):982–9. https://doi.org/10.1164/rccm.200603-344OC.
19. Makris D, Scherpereel A, Leroy S, et al. Electromagnetic navigation diagnostic bronchoscopy for small peripheral lung lesions. Eur Respir J. 2007;29(6):1187–92. https://doi.org/10.1183/09031936.00165306.
20. Eberhardt R, Anantham D, Ernst A, et al. Multimodality bronchoscopic diagnosis of peripheral lung lesions: a randomized controlled trial. Am J Respir Crit Care Med. 2007;176(1):36–41. https://doi.org/10.1164/rccm.200612-1866OC.
21. Kumar M, Shanavas M, Sidappa A, et al. Cone beam computed tomography - know its secrets. J Int Oral Health. 2015;7(2):64–8.
22. Folch EE, Bowling MR, Pritchett MA, et al. NAVIGATE 24-month results: electromagnetic navigation bronchoscopy for pulmonary lesions at 37 centers in Europe and the United States. J Thorac Oncol. 2022;17(4):519–31. https://doi.org/10.1016/j.jtho.2021.12.008.
23. Duke JD, Reisenauer J. Review: technology and techniques for robotic-assisted bronchoscopy. J Lung Health Dis. 2022;6(1):1–5.
24. Chaddha U, Kovacs SP, Manley C, et al. Robot-assisted bronchoscopy for pulmonary lesion diagnosis: results from the initial multicenter experience. BMC Pulm Med. 2019;19(1):243. https://doi.org/10.1186/s12890-019-1010-8.
25. Anantham D, Feller-Kopman D, Shanmugham LN, et al. Electromagnetic navigation bronchoscopy-guided fiducial placement for robotic stereotactic radiosurgery of lung tumors: a feasibility study. Chest. 2007;132(3):930–5. https://doi.org/10.1378/chest.07-0522.
26. Loddenkemper R, Praveen NM, Noppen M. Medical thoracoscopy/pleuroscopy: manual and atlas. Thieme; 2010.
27. Strong MS, Jako GJ, Polanyi T, et al. Laser surgery in the aerodigestive tract. Am J Surg. 1973;126(4):529–33. https://doi.org/10.1016/s0002-9610(73)80044-3.
28. Dumon JF, Reboud E, Auconte F, et al. Treatment of tracheobronchial lesions with Laser Yag. Minerva Med. 1981;72(39):2593–600.
29. Dumon JF, Reboud E, Garbe L, et al. Treatment of tracheobronchial lesions by laser photoresection. Chest. 1982;81(3):278–84. https://doi.org/10.1378/chest.81.3.278.
30. Lee P, Kupeli E, Mehta AC. Therapeutic bronchoscopy in lung cancer. Laser therapy, electrocautery, brachytherapy, stents, and photodynamic therapy. Clin Chest Med. 2002;23(1):241–56. https://doi.org/10.1016/s0272-5231(03)00075-3.
31. Moghissi K, Dixon K. Bronchoscopic NdYAG laser treatment in lung cancer, 30 years on: an institutional review. Lasers Med Sci. 2006;21(4):186–91. https://doi.org/10.1007/s10103-006-0400-3.

32. Sutedja T, et al. Endobronchial electrocautery is an excellent alternative for Nd:YAG laser to treat airway tumors. J Bronchology Interv Pulmonol. 1997;4:101–5.
33. De la Cruz LI, Pereira A, Krieger B. Use of endobronchial electrocautery for the palliation of airway obstruction due to metastases from nonpulmonary malignancies. J Bronchol. 2006;13(3):124–7.
34. Reichle G, Freitag L, Kullmann HJ, et al. [Argon plasma coagulation in bronchology: a new method--alternative or complementary?]. Pneumologie. 2000;54(11):508–16. https://doi.org/10.1055/s-2000-8254.
35. Reddy C, Majid A, Michaud G, et al. Gas embolism following bronchoscopic argon plasma coagulation: a case series. Chest. 2008;134(5):1066–9. https://doi.org/10.1378/chest.08-0474.
36. Interventions in pulmonary medicine. Springer Nature Switzerland AG. 2023.
37. Lund ME, Force S. Airway stenting for patients with benign airway disease and the Food and Drug Administration advisory: a call for restraint. Chest. 2007;132(4):1107–8. https://doi.org/10.1378/chest.07-0242.
38. Rodriguez AN, Díaz-Jiménez JP, Edell ES. Silicone stents versus metal stents for management of benign tracheobronchial disease con: metal stents. J Bronchol Interv Pulmonol. 2000;7(2):184–7.
39. Wood DE. Airway stenting. Chest Surg Clin N Am. 2001;11(4):841–60.
40. Jantz MA, Silvestri GA. Silicone stents versus metal stents for management of benign tracheobronchial disease pro: metal stents. J Bronchol. 2000;7(2):177–83.
41. Criner GJ, Sue R, Wright S, et al. A multicenter randomized controlled trial of Zephyr endobronchial valve treatment in heterogeneous emphysema (LIBERATE). Am J Respir Crit Care Med. 2018;198(9):1151–64. https://doi.org/10.1164/rccm.201803-0590OC.
42. Colt HG, Morris JF. Fiberoptic bronchoscopy without premedication. A retrospective study. Chest. 1990;98(6):1327–30. https://doi.org/10.1378/chest.98.6.1327.
43. Hatton MQ, Allen MB, Vathenen AS, et al. Does sedation help in fibreoptic bronchoscopy? BMJ. 1994;309(6963):1206–7. https://doi.org/10.1136/bmj.309.6963.1206.
44. Ni YL, Lo YL, Lin TY, et al. Conscious sedation reduces patient discomfort and improves satisfaction in flexible bronchoscopy. Chang Gung Med J. 2010;33(4):443–52.
45. Stolz D, Kurer G, Meyer A, et al. Propofol versus combined sedation in flexible bronchoscopy: a randomised non-inferiority trial. Eur Respir J. 2009;34(5):1024–30. https://doi.org/10.1183/09031936.00180808.
46. Goudra BG, Singh PM, Borle A, et al. Anesthesia for advanced bronchoscopic procedures: state-of-the-art review. Lung. 2015;193(4):453–65. https://doi.org/10.1007/s00408-015-9733-7.
47. Maguire GP, Rubinfeld AR, Trembath PW, et al. Patients prefer sedation for fibreoptic bronchoscopy. Respirology. 1998;3(2):81–5. https://doi.org/10.1111/j.1440-1843.1998.tb00101.x.
48. Prakash UB, Offord KP, Stubbs SE. Bronchoscopy in North America: the ACCP survey. Chest. 1991;100(6):1668–75. https://doi.org/10.1378/chest.100.6.1668.
49. Gaisl T, Bratton DJ, Heuss LT, et al. Sedation during bronchoscopy: data from a nationwide sedation and monitoring survey. BMC Pulm Med. 2016;16(1):113. https://doi.org/10.1186/s12890-016-0275-4.
50. Simon M, Braune S, Frings D, et al. High-flow nasal cannula oxygen versus non-invasive ventilation in patients with acute hypoxaemic respiratory failure undergoing flexible bronchoscopy--a prospective randomised trial. Crit Care. 2014;18(6):712. https://doi.org/10.1186/s13054-014-0712-9.
51. Emerson C, Ali A. Airway management for subglottic stenting. Paediatr Anaesth. 2010;20(1):114. https://doi.org/10.1111/j.1460-9592.2009.03220.x.
52. Sastre JA, Cordovilla R, Jiménez MF, et al. Management of a transbronchial cryobiopsy using the i-gel® airway and the Arndt endobronchial blocker. Can J Anaesth. 2014;61(9):886–8. https://doi.org/10.1007/s12630-014-0191-0.
53. Slebos DJ, Shah PL, Herth FJ, et al. Endobronchial valves for endoscopic lung volume reduction: best practice recommendations from expert panel on endoscopic lung volume reduction. Respiration. 2017;93(2):138–50. https://doi.org/10.1159/000453588.

54. Sarkiss M. Anesthesia for bronchoscopy and interventional pulmonology: from moderate sedation to jet ventilation. Curr Opin Pulm Med. 2011;17(4):274–8. https://doi.org/10.1097/MCP.0b013e3283471227.
55. Wu SH, Lu DV, Hsu CD, et al. The effectiveness of low-dose dexmedetomidine infusion in sedative flexible bronchoscopy: a retrospective analysis. Medicina (Kaunas). 2020;56(4):193. https://doi.org/10.3390/medicina56040193.
56. Pertzov B, Krasulya B, Azem K, et al. Dexmedetomidine versus propofol sedation in flexible bronchoscopy: a randomized controlled trial. BMC Pulm Med. 2022;22(1):87. https://doi.org/10.1186/s12890-022-01880-9.
57. Banerjee S, McCormack S. Ketamine for sedation during bronchoscopy procedures: a review of clinical effectiveness, safety, and guidelines. 2020.
58. Galway U, Zura A, Khanna S, et al. Anesthetic considerations for bronchoscopic procedures: a narrative review based on the Cleveland Clinic experience. J Thorac Dis. 2019;11(7):3156–70. https://doi.org/10.21037/jtd.2019.07.29.
59. Magnusson L, Spahn DR. New concepts of atelectasis during general anaesthesia. Br J Anaesth. 2003;91(1):61–72. https://doi.org/10.1093/bja/aeg085.
60. Abdelmalak BB, Gildea TR, Doyle DJ. Anesthesia for bronchoscopy. Curr Pharm Des. 2012;18(38):6314–24. https://doi.org/10.2174/138161212803832290.
61. Clark G, Licker M, Younossian AB, et al. Titrated sedation with propofol or midazolam for flexible bronchoscopy: a randomised trial. Eur Respir J. 2009;34(6):1277–83. https://doi.org/10.1183/09031936.00142108.
62. Avidan MS, Zhang L, Burnside BA, et al. Anesthesia awareness and the bispectral index. N Engl J Med. 2008;358(11):1097–108. https://doi.org/10.1056/NEJMoa0707361.

Preoperative Assessment and Optimization

2

Angela Roberts Selzer and Benjamin H. Cloyd

2.1 Introduction

The preanesthesia evaluation is an opportunity to elucidate the patient's underlying medical disease, determine if the patient is optimized, treat modifiable conditions, screen for potentially unrecognized disorders, and assess overall risk for perioperative complications. Relative to their nonevaluated peers, patients who have a thorough preoperative evaluation in a preanesthesia clinic have been shown to have reduced same-day case delays and cancellations [1, 2], decreased hospital length of stays (hLOS) [3], and a reduction in in-hospital mortality rates [4].

In this chapter, we will be presenting the principles of a thorough preoperative assessment and preoperative optimization plan for interventional pulmonology (IP) patients. We will cover the general principles of preoperative assessment, with a specific emphasis on optimizing patients with pulmonary disease. We will also detail the components of a thorough airway exam and discuss how to utilize this assessment to create a safe anesthetic plan.

IP procedures are never *truly elective* procedures, and this must be taken into consideration when performing a periprocedural risk assessment for patients. Patients deemed too high risk to undergo thoracic surgery, for example, may be offered an IP procedure as a lower risk "nonsurgical" alternative diagnostic or therapeutic intervention. While IP procedures *are* less invasive than surgery, the inherent risks of general anesthesia and the implications of a shared and/or difficult airway need to be taken into account, especially in a patient population with pulmonary disease.

Patients scheduled to undergo IP procedures should be screened for evaluation in a preanesthesia clinic, where the patient can be assessed for fitness for anesthesia and modifiable risk factors can be addressed and treated, such as anemia, smoking,

A. R. Selzer (✉) · B. H. Cloyd
University of Colorado School of Medicine, Anschutz Medical Campus, Aurora, CO, USA
e-mail: Angela.Selzer@cuanschutz.edu; Benjamin.Cloyd@cuanschutz.edu

M. Sarkiss (ed.), *Anesthesia for Interventional Pulmonary Procedures*,
https://doi.org/10.1007/978-3-032-12007-6_2

deconditioning, and malnutrition. These interventions have been shown to improve outcomes but can take significant time to accomplish (from 4 to 8 weeks) and must be balanced with the risks of delaying procedures, as there can also be significant risks associated with delay. Delays in *diagnostic* procedures can result in treatment delays and worsened outcomes. Whereas, delays in *therapeutic* procedures can result in worsened outcomes due to functional disability and continued cardiopulmonary stress.

Therefore, the preanesthetic assessment of IP patients should seek to provide a thoughtful, thorough assessment that accounts for procedural urgency and balances the risks of delay with potential benefits of optimizing underlying comorbidities.

2.2 General Preanesthesia Assessment

The major components of a preanesthesia evaluation include a physical exam, history taking, risk assessment, laboratory testing, and imaging.

2.2.1 Physical Exam

A thorough physical exam performed during the preoperative clinic visit can guide testing and determine the presence and severity of a patient's underlying comorbidities. A basic physical exam includes height and weight, blood pressure, pulse oximetry, and respiratory rate. All patients presenting for a preanesthesia evaluation should have thorough cardiopulmonary and airway exams. Other aspects of the physical exam should be guided by the medical history, chief complaint, and review of systems.

Patients presenting for a biopsy of suspected malignancy should be examined for lymphadenopathy. Presence of an easily palpable node may alter diagnostic planning and should be discussed with the oncologic team. Patients presenting for biopsy of mediastinal masses should be examined for worrisome signs of superior vena cava (SVC) syndrome. Findings on physical exam have important implications on anesthetic planning as they are high risk for a cannot-ventilate, cannot-intubate scenario in the operating room (discussed below). Signs of SVC syndrome include facial swelling, upper extremity swelling, distended jugular veins, horseness, or wheezing. Patients should be placed in the supine position to see if this elicits symptoms and oxygenation measured with a pulse oximeter.

2.2.2 Cardiopulmonary Exam

Auscultation of the heart and lungs, while basic skills of any clinician, should not be underestimated in their ability to impact the preoperative assessment of patients. While IP patients have almost certainly had lung auscultation performed in their pulmonologist's office, underlying diseases such as chronic obstructive pulmonary disease (COPD), pulmonary hypertension (PH), and central airway obstructions (CAO) are dynamic processes. Findings such as crackles, wheezing, and decreased breath sounds can impact preanesthetic planning, warranting delay or, alternatively, increasing the urgency of the proposed procedure. Unexpected or worrisome pulmonary exam findings should be compared to another documented clinician exam and a follow-up approach developed with a multidisciplinary team, including the interventional pulmonologist and primary care provider.

The absence or presence of additional findings consistent with chronic hypoxia should be documented, including digital clubbing and central, peripheral, or mixed cyanosis. Signs of right ventricular (RV) heart failure are particularly worrisome in patients with chronic pulmonary disease as they indicate decompensated pulmonary hypertension. Cool, pale digits with prolonged capillary refill time, distended jugular veins, hepatomegaly, ascites, and peripheral edema are all signs of RV failure [5].

A murmur heard on exam not explained by a known cardiac diagnosis warrants obtaining an echocardiogram to rule out valvular disease, left ventricular outflow tract obstruction, or a patent foramen ovale [6]. All of these conditions have important implications on both anesthetic and long-term management. Testing is discussed in more detail later in the chapter. Experienced clinicians may appreciate an accentuated pulmonary component of the second heart sound, and an RV third heart sound may also be present.

2.2.3 Airway Exam

The preoperative airway assessment of patients undergoing IP procedures aims to preemptively identify issues that may compromise the ability to safely and effectively oxygenate and ventilate the patient, or the ability to safely perform the procedure itself. Similar to otolaryngologic surgery, IP procedures mandate a "shared airway" between the anesthesiologist and pulmonologist, and thus require a shared understanding of each patient's physiologic, anatomic, and procedural-specific considerations [7]. As patients undergoing IP procedures will often have pathologic conditions that may generate both physiologically and anatomically challenging airway management conditions, a structured, detailed preoperative airway assessment, plan, and overarching strategy are essential as the possibility of rapid oxygen desaturation and its subsequent consequences in these patients should not be underestimated. With a primary focus on patient safety and optimal clinical outcomes, we present a framework to evaluate a patient's upper and lower (central) airways, along with special situations, which merit additional attention from the anesthesia team, including aspiration risk, preoperative extubation planning considerations, and veno-venous extracorporeal membrane oxygenation (VV ECMO) support. We note that in this section we focus primarily on the preoperative considerations related to airway management, and intraprocedural and postprocedural airway considerations will be discussed elsewhere.

We caution that no single assessment strategy, tool, or anesthetic technique can be universally relied upon for IP (or any anesthetic) cases, and each case requires an individualized, adaptable plan [8]. Again, similarly to otolaryngologic surgery, preoperative planning should focus on identifying the right place, timing, and personnel needed to produce a step-wise strategy of primary and backup plans to ensure the best outcome [7]. A preoperative airway examination should consider as much information as is reasonably available to the anesthesiologist and is ideally performed in a multidisciplinary fashion with consultation available to a diverse team, including the interventional pulmonologist, to consider procedure-specific issues.

In addition to evaluating for external anatomic predictors of upper airway management difficulty, the anesthesia team should evaluate the most recent available radiologic imaging, prior anesthetic, and procedural notes, along with any bronchoscopic findings when available. We also note that recent efforts to improve airway management safety have appropriately directed more attention to the "physiologically difficult airway," defined as one in which physiologic alterations increase the risk for cardiorespiratory and other complications during tracheal intubation and the transition to positive pressure ventilation, a situation that is commonly encountered during IP procedures [9].

2.2.3.1 Preoperative Airway Evaluation Techniques

Every preprocedural airway assessment for any anesthetic should include a structured evaluation of the face and the upper airway. There are multiple widely used airway assessment techniques and strategies, each with its own strengths and weaknesses. A complete review of these is not possible here, though we recommend utilizing a consistent, structured method, which simultaneously evaluates and gives weight to multiple anatomic predictors, while also considering the patients' current and future physiologic state, along with the context in which the airway management decision is being made. At minimum, we recommend evaluating several key components, including a Mallampati score, thyromental distance, mouth opening and inter-incisor gap, presence of beard, dentition, upper lip bite test, tongue size, neck circumference, neck flexion and extension, and a history of obstructive sleep apnea or head and neck radiation (Table 2.1). Of note, even with a thorough and reassuring preoperative airway assessment, difficulty in management may still occur. A 2015 Danish study found that 93% of difficult intubations were unanticipated, along with 94% of cases of difficult mask ventilation [10]. With this concern of unpredictability in mind, a strategy for managing airway difficulty should always be in place [11].

Table 2.1 Components of a basic preprocedural airway exam

Mallampati score	Neck circumference
Thyromental distance	Neck flexion
Mouth opening	Neck extension
Inter-incisor gap	Presence of facial hair
Quality of dentition	History of or risk for obstructive sleep apnea
Upper lip bite test	History of head and neck surgery
Tongue size	History of head and neck radiation

The Canadian Airway Focus Group (CAFG) employs a more inclusive definition of "difficult airway" than other societies, which often tend to focus on issues with predicted anatomic difficulty [12]. The CAFG recognizes a difficult airway as one where an experienced airway manager anticipates or encounters difficulty with any or all of laryngoscopy or tracheal intubation, face-mask ventilation (FMV), supraglottic airway (SGA) use, or emergent front of neck access (eFONA) [12]. They note that the airway extends from the nostrils and lips to the alveoli, and anatomical variation or pathological distortion anywhere along its length may cause difficulty, and context may compound difficulty as well [12]. At least one or even all of these issues is often present in patients requiring IP procedures, and the patient with a previously known or predicted anatomically "difficult airway" presents a special challenge in the IP suite, and even greater consideration should be given to preoperative airway planning in this patient population. With these issues in mind, strong consideration should be given to awake intubation techniques when clinically indicated.

The choice of an endotracheal tube, LMA, rigid bronchoscope, tubeless field, or other airway management device depends on both patient needs and procedural requirements. When not contraindicated, LMAs provide the benefit of being both less stimulating and enhanced access to the proceduralist of proximal airway structures [13]. When tracheal intubation is being considered or required, video laryngoscopy provides the benefit that all parties are able to see and evaluate the upper airways, and confirm appropriate location of ideal tube placement. Recent high-quality evidence has demonstrated that the use of video laryngoscopy is associated with improved first-pass success [14, 15]. As patients undergoing IP procedures often have anatomically difficult airways coupled with physiologic issues that may make first-pass success paramount, we recommend that whenever possible video laryngoscopy be used as the preferred first choice for tracheal intubation when awake tracheal intubation is not indicated, or that a video laryngoscope be immediately available, which is supported by numerous clinical recommendations and guidelines [15–17].

IP airway management difficulty is also often compounded by pathology in the central and lower airways, which may prevent tube passage or gas exchange. Patients undergoing IP procedures may have relatively simple tracheal tube or LMA placement, but effective oxygenation and ventilation may subsequently become impossible following induction of anesthesia or intubation [18]. With this in mind, careful preanesthetic evaluation of the central and lower airways with a multidisciplinary team, including the pulmonologist, is essential. The patient's most recently available radiologic examinations, including chest radiographs and CT scans when available, should be reviewed whenever possible [17, 18].

Central airway obstruction (CAO), in particular, is a life-threatening problem that is one of the most challenging pathologies facing anesthesiologists and is associated with a poor prognosis [18]. CAO is defined as a 50% or greater occlusion of the trachea, mainstem bronchi, bronchus intermedius, or lobar bronchi [18, 19]. Lung cancer is the most common cause of malignant CAO, but it can also be caused by primary airway malignancies, metastases to the airway or surrounding mediastinum, or nonmalignant disorders. CAO itself is classified into three anatomic categories: intrinsic, extrinsic, or mixed [18, 19]. As discussed later in this chapter, patients with CAO should be considered for alternative means of airway management, including ECMO.

Finally, when available, it can be beneficial to evaluate prior anesthetic records for insights into whether there were issues with initial airway management, ventilation, or other relevant anesthetic concerns. However, an individualized evaluation and overarching strategy is necessitated for each encounter based on the current needs of the patient and the proposed procedure as both patient-specific issues and procedural needs may change.

2.2.3.2 Aspiration Considerations

Pulmonary aspiration remains a leading cause of anesthesia morbidity and mortality, and every patient undergoing sedation or a general anesthetic should have an evaluation of their aspiration risk and appropriate steps taken to mitigate that risk if possible. Though rare, aspiration is ten times more common than a cannot-intubate, cannot-oxygenate scenario, and is particularly devastating to patients with preexisting pulmonary conditions [20]. Patients with a full stomach or any full stomach equivalent should be intubated [17]. Specific to patients undergoing interventional pulmonary procedures are anatomic derangements that can place them at a higher risk of aspiration, even when appropriately fasted, including tracheo-esophageal fistulas and friable airway lesions. If known, the location and size of fistulas, lesions, or other pathologies should be reviewed on the preoperative chest CT, and the plans for airway management, method of ventilation, and methods of rescue should be discussed and agreed upon among the entire care team prior to the procedure [17].

Given the risk that aspiration presents to IP patients, a multimodal method to prevent it or its consequences should it occur should be employed with every anesthetic. A complete review of aspiration prevention and management has significant nuance and is beyond the scope of this chapter, but we in general recommend making efforts to prevent aspiration via appropriate fasting times, pharmacologic prophylaxis when indicated, consideration of awake intubation or rapid sequence induction, and the immediate availability of the tools and equipment necessary to mitigate or manage the impact of pulmonary aspiration should it occur. Emerging techniques such as gastric ultrasound are developing to evaluate whether patients have gastric contents visible on ultrasound. Though they have yet to be extensively incorporated into practice and guidelines, we believe, given ultrasound's low threshold to perform and lack of risk to the patient, it is reasonable to utilize gastric ultrasound as one element in a constellation of tools when evaluating a patient's perioperative aspiration risk, similar to airway risk assessment. Finally, we caution that it has been consistently noted that half, if not more, of aspiration episodes occur outside the time of anesthetic induction, and that continuous vigilance, along with methods to both reduce the risk and manage aspiration, should be employed throughout the perioperative period [20].

2.2.3.3 Preoperative Extubation Considerations

Extubation planning begins with preoperative planning. While traditionally less attention has focused on failed tracheal extubation compared to failed tracheal intubation, evidence has demonstrated that a significant proportion of airway-related issues occur at extubation, including the ASA Closed Claims Database, along with the Fourth National Audit Project (NAP4), which found that a quarter of airway-related morbidity and mortality occurred post extubation [21, 22]. With this knowledge in mind, the Difficult Airway Society (DAS) developed a set of tracheal extubation guidelines that provide excellent strategies to evaluate, prepare for, and subsequently manage both low-risk and at-risk tracheal extubations [23]. When first evaluating a patient for an IP procedure, special attention should be given to the patient and procedural characteristics, along with the contextual issues that will dictate the patient's chances at a successful extubation.

An "at-risk" extubation as described by the DAS is a common scenario in the IP patient population as they often have some, if not all, of the complicating factors that contribute to a high-risk extubation, including anatomic, physiologic, and contextual concerns. These issues may worsen postoperatively as a result of the procedure, including airway swelling or bleeding, compounded by residual sedation, neuromuscular weakness, and/or other physiologic derangements [23]. Considering this, an evaluation of a patient's suitability for extubation should consider both the preoperative airway evaluation characteristics predictive of difficulty, and those that may change during the procedure (including changes to airway anatomy) that would dictate whether they may be difficult to reintubate [10–12].

Patients at high risk for extubation failure or with other possible needs for postoperative ventilatory support should have their procedure performed in a facility with immediate, on-site access to intensive care services. Finally, we note the patient and procedural characteristics specific to IP procedures associated with failed extubation, along with strategies to improve or mitigate these concerns, are currently underexplored and merit further study.

2.2.3.4 ECMO Considerations

In cases where there is significant concern for a cannot-intubate, cannot-ventilate or oxygenate scenario, the patient may be best managed with extracorporeal oxygenation support, most likely by VV ECMO [13]. This approach can provide oxygenation while attempts to secure a definitive airway or perform the procedure are carried out in a controlled environment [24]. As per the American College of Chest Physicians clinical guidelines, the use of ECMO should be considered in patients with severe (or near-complete) airway obstruction secondary to anterior neck or tracheal disease [18]. A 2015 single-center review of 15 cases requiring ECMO for upper airway surgery recommended that evidence of tracheal patency less than 5 mm should prompt consideration of elective cannulae insertion [25].

Ideally, cases that may require VV ECMO should be identified as early as possible, and an appropriate multidisciplinary discussion should be held, including anesthesiologists who regularly perform these techniques, and plans made for the timing and location of the procedure to ensure adequate access to advanced therapies. Calling for ECMO when the patient is already in a cannot-intubate, cannot-oxygenate scenario is generally too late and should be avoided whenever possible. A 2009 meta-analysis found a nearly two times greater risk of mortality when ECMO was not initiated within 30 minutes of cardiac arrest, and that the average time from the beginning of CPR to initiation of ECMO was approximately 40 minutes, highlighting the difficulty of initiating this intervention [26]. We again note that in our experience, even under controlled, semi-elective conditions, the initiation of ECMO support is complex and technically challenging and should be planned as far in advance as reasonably possible. When utilized in a controlled fashion, ECMO support can provide a safe method for airway management in patients where other methods may be impossible and has been shown to yield excellent surgical conditions and, more importantly, good patient outcomes [24].

2.2.4 Testing

Patients without significant systemic disease undergoing low-risk procedures should proceed without any testing, regardless of age. Reducing routine preoperative laboratory testing, cardiac testing, and chest radiographs is a significant source of unnecessary testing and the focus of the American Board of Internal Medicine (ABIM) Choosing Wisely Campaign (http://www.choosingwisely.org/) [27]. Therefore, unlike for thoracic surgery patients, there is no *routine* serum laboratory testing that need be done prior to IP procedures. A patient without severe systemic disease and no recent changes in overall health need not undergo routine testing prior to an IP procedure even if no testing has been performed since their last annual exam.

Unfortunately, the majority of IP patients *have* either severe systemic disease and/or recent changes in overall health. It is not uncommon to see laboratory abnormalities in this patient population. Hypokalemia, hyponatremia, anemia, neutropenia, and/or thrombocytopenia can be seen in patients with a diagnosed or suspected malignancy. Patients with severe pulmonary disease and/or malnutrition may also have electrolyte abnormalities that should be followed closely and treated. Patients with COPD and/or chronic hypoxia may have erythrocytosis. In these patients, baseline testing of a complete blood count (CBC) and basic metabolic panel (BMP) is clinically suggested.

Fortunately, most IP patients will have had some degree of testing performed prior to referral to the preoperative clinic. These should be reviewed, and repeat testing considered based on a review of systems. With recent *normal* laboratory values, no additional testing need be done. The definition of recent testing varies by institution (at our institution, we use testing within 60 days). However, these definitions are arbitrary and lack consensus within the perioperative medicine community. Clinical judgment should be used to determine if labs need be drawn more or less frequently. It is reasonable in an otherwise healthy patient to find normal testing within a year acceptable.

Other chronic diseases may warrant additional testing. For example, a baseline creatinine in a hypertensive patient [28]. The preanesthesia clinic also presents an additional opportunity to perform necessary screening tests when warranted. The American Diabetes Association recommends screening for diabetes in patients with risk factors for diabetes and for all patients over the age of 35 with an HgbA1C [29]. Screening for diabetes in patients who have, for various reasons, not had access to this test may have lifelong implications on morbidity and mortality. Additional testing can be considered based on findings during a review of systems.

While routine chest radiography is not recommended by the American College of Radiology [27], most, if not all, IP patients have had radiographs, computed tomography (CT), and/or magnetic resonance imaging (MRI) studies performed. These should be reviewed and may reveal underlying lung pathology. Low oxygen saturation, lung findings on exam, or a positive review of symptoms may also trigger additional workup [30].

Routine electrocardiography (ECG) screening is not indicated in asymptomatic patients. However, many IP patients have smoking histories and other risk factors for ischemic heart disease. An ECG to screen for ischemic heart disease in elevated-risk patients with low functional status is reasonable if there is no recent ECG (which we define as within 1 year). Further testing is discussed in the cardiovascular risk assessment. The ECG is cost-effective and typically the best first step for workup of any new cardiopulmonary findings on physical exam.

Left ventricular function should be assessed in patients reporting new dyspnea or findings consistent with heart failure. This is a grade 1 recommendation by the 2024 ACC/AHA/HRS Guideline of Perioperative Cardiovascular Management for Non-Cardiac Surgery [6]. Additionally, they make a grade 1 recommendation to perform echocardiography in any patient with suspected moderate-to-severe valvular disease [6]. The ACC/AHA 2020 Guideline for the Management of Patients with Valvular Heart Disease recommends routine scheduled screening in patients with known valvular disease based on severity and location of disease [31]. It is important to ensure that this recommended surveillance is completed to avoid the risk of inducing general anesthesia in a patient with severe or critical disease.

Routine pulmonary function testing (PFT) is also not indicated in patients undergoing IP procedures. It is important to ensure that patients are compliant with the recommendations of their pulmonologist and have completed testing as per their most recent pulmonology visit. Being due or overdue for repeat PFTs is the most common reason we facilitate this test in our preanesthetic clinic. Many IP patients will have had PFTs recently performed. It is worthwhile to review these and summarize this information for the anesthetic team to tailor their anesthetic plan. Patients with very poor function on PFT (FEV1 and/or DLCO <30% expected) may be particularly difficult to wean from the ventilator postprocedurally. A discussion of postanesthetic planning and possible admission for extended ventilation is important to have with the patient and pulmonologist before the scheduled procedure. Advanced care planning wishes are discussed in more detail later in this chapter.

A six-minute walk distance (6MWD) is a test that is cheap to perform and can readily identify patients with severe pulmonary disease who are at elevated risk for pulmonary complications after anesthetics. Prior values in 6MWD can provide context into a patient's current state of health, effectiveness of therapy, or need for additional treatment. A 6MWD <325 meters predicts postoperative pulmonary complications with 77% sensitivity and 100% specificity [32].

2.2.5 Functional Assessment

Patients who can achieve an activity level of ≥4 Metabolic Equivalents of Task (METs) *without* symptoms do not require further cardiopulmonary testing to undergo low-risk, nonvascular surgery [33] (1 MET = 3.5 mL O2 consumption/kg of body weight/min). In patients who do not perform traditional exercise, they may meet this four MET threshold of energy expenditure while performing routine household activities such as strenuous housework, mowing one's lawn or walking up a flight of stairs [34]. The Duke Activity Scale Index (DASI) is another method of functional assessment [35]. Cardiopulmonary testing with VO2 measurement is the gold standard for functional testing but is uncommonly utilized in the United States.

Mobility issues with many IP patients can make evaluating their cardiopulmonary fitness challenging. In patients with a limited functional status, it is unknown whether they have adequate cardiovascular fitness to tolerate the stress of general anesthesia. In patients who either cannot achieve four METs or who are symptomatic at that level of activity, the ACC/AHA/ASE/ASNC/HFSA/HRS/SCAI/SCCT/SCMR/STS 2024 Appropriate Use Criteria for Multimodality Imaging in Cardiovascular Evaluation of Patients Undergoing Nonemergent, Noncardiac Surgery [33] can help guide additional cardiovascular testing, described in more detail in the cardiac risk assessment section.

2.2.6 Risk Assessments

While a comprehensive risk assessment is a key component of a thorough pre-anesthesia assessment, there are no validated risk assessment tools for patients scheduled to undergo IP procedures. Among others, there are cardiac, pulmonary, and venous thromboembolism risk tools that have been validated in surgical patient populations. Additionally, appropriate use criteria for testing do not specifically address periprocedural risk. While it is reasonable to use these tools to extrapolate from the low-risk surgical population to procedural patients, it is important to note that they have not been validated in this patient population. However, the highest risk patients are subjected to for most low-risk surgical procedures is the risk of general anesthesia. The same may be said for interventional procedures as well. Therefore, at our institution, we choose the low-risk nonvascular surgical procedure to be an acceptable approximation of procedural risk. Table 2.2 summarizes the commonly utilized risk assessment and screening tools.

Table 2.2 Common perioperative screening and risk assessment tools

Tool	Use
Gupta MICA risk calculator [37]	Perioperative cardiac risk calculator
ACS-SRC [38]	American College of Surgery Surgical Risk Calculator
Caprini score [42]	Perioperative VTE risk
Ariscat score [41]	Postoperative Pulmonary Risk Calculator
STOP-BANG [47]	OSA Screening Tool
Frailty index [53]	Frailty Scoring Tool
PONS score [55]	Perioperative Malnutrition Screening Tool

MICA myocardial infarction or cardiac arrest, *VTE* venous thromboembolism, *OSA* obstructive sleep apnea, *PONS* perioperative nutrition screening

The most widely validated cardiac risk assessment tool, the modified RCRI has fallen out of favor due to its development prior to the advent of minimally invasive surgical techniques [36]. There are a number of newer cardiac risk calculators used and validated that require the use of an online calculator to perform. The Gupta Index, published in 2011, assesses the risk for perioperative myocardial infarction (MI) and cardiac arrest (CA) [37]. It was developed from the 2007 National Surgical Quality Improvement Program (NSQIP) database and included 211,410 patients. It is the calculator of choice in our institution.

The American College of Surgeons (ACS) developed an online Surgical Risk Calculator (SRC) that assesses individual risk for 12 different adverse events, including cardiac [38, 39]. This was also derived from the NSQIP database from 2009 to 2012 and included 1,414,006 patients. Use of the ACS-SRC requires knowledge of the patient's specific surgery (as designated by one of 1557 CPT codes) and entry of 19 specific patient factors. While somewhat cumbersome to use, it is useful because it evaluates risk for 12 complications and provides patients with a visual representation of their relative risk of complications compared to an average patient having the same surgery. Risk of death or discharge to nursing or rehab facility are outcomes of particular interest to patients, and it is worthwhile for surgeons to display the ACS-SRC table when obtaining informed surgical consent.

Both the Gupta Index and the ACS-SRC require selection of either a surgical specialty or CPT code. If utilizing a cardiac risk factor would contribute to the assessment of the IP patient, it is reasonable to consider selecting a low-risk surgical procedure (e.g., laparoscopic appendectomy) with the caveat that the results will be a gross estimate of individual risk relative to average but not specific to procedural risk.

In patients with poor or unknown functional capacity and no other cardiac risk modifiers, these cardiac risk assessments help guide cardiovascular testing [6]. In these patients with an elevated risk of perioperative myocardial events (>1%), the ACC/AHA/HRS guidelines for perioperative cardiovascular management for noncardiac surgery recommend (grade 2a) screening with cardiac biomarker assessment, namely, brain-natriuretic peptide (BNP) or N-terminal pro-B-type natriuretic peptide (NT-proBNP) [6]. Significant cardiac disease can be essentially ruled out with normal biomarkers, whereas abnormal biomarkers should warrant further investigation and multidisciplinary conversation.

Cardiac risk assessment tools tend to underestimate risk in patients with conditions that are known to increase perioperative risk but are not included in cardiac risk calculators, for example, pulmonary hypertension or congenital heart disease. The 2024 guidelines address this concern by describing comorbidities considered "risk-modifiers" that include severe valvular heart disease, severe pulmonary hypertension, elevated risk congenital heart disease, prior coronary stents, prior coronary bypass surgery, recent stroke, implanted pacemaker, implanted defibrillator, and/or frailty [6]. In these patients, ECG (grade 2A) and echocardiography (grade 1/2A) should be considered. Additionally, patients should be following goal-directed medical therapy (GDMT) and established testing guidelines for their specific conditions.

Extrapolating recommendations for low-risk, nonvascular surgery to IP procedures means that preprocedural cardiovascular imaging is rarely indicated in this patient population. As described previously, it is unnecessary to perform cardiopulmonary testing on patients who can achieve four METs without symptoms [33]. However, it is reasonable to obtain a transthoracic echocardiogram (TTE) in patients unable to achieve four METs without symptoms *and* with known or suspected valvular heart disease *without* recent cardiovascular imaging (within 220 days). It is also reasonable to obtain a TTE and/or stress testing in patients unable to achieve four METs without symptoms *and* with known or suspected ischemic heart disease *without* recent cardiovascular imaging (within 220 days). In patients unable to achieve four METs without symptoms *and* with known or suspected heart disease *with* recent abnormal stress testing, it is reasonable to consider a TTE before low-risk, nonvascular surgery.

Ultimately, IP procedures tend to be both nonelective and time-sensitive. The timely ability to obtain cardiovascular imaging, including a TTE or stress testing, can assist the anesthesia team in the careful anesthetic planning and management. However, the risk–benefit of coronary revascularization to reduce perioperative cardiac risk should take into account the patient's long-term prognosis and the risks of delaying pulmonary intervention to proceed with coronary intervention first. These are complex decisions that should be made in a multidisciplinary fashion, including pulmonology, cardiology, and anesthesiology while also centering shared decision-making with the patient.

Postoperative pulmonary complications (PPCs) occur as frequently as cardiac complications and result in increased costs, morbidity, and long-term mortality [40]. There are several pulmonary risk calculators that have been validated in surgical, but not procedural, patients. We use the ARISCAT pulmonary risk calculator at our institution [41]. An important feature of the ARISCAT calculator is that it predicts the likelihood of any PPC, including pneumonia, respiratory failure, pleural effusion, atelectasis, pneumothorax, bronchospasm, and aspiration pneumonitis. Patients in the highest risk group of this index have a 44% risk of PPCs. Age, preoperative SpO2, respiratory infection within 1 month, anemia, surgical incision site, duration of surgery, and emergency surgery are the predictors used in the model.

Patients are at an increased risk of venous thromboembolism (VTE) in the perioperative period due to venous stasis, inflammation, reduced mobility, and a hypercoagulable state. Again, we do not have data to determine if a similar risk exists in periprocedural patients. However, venous stasis and reduced mobility are common to all patients who undergo a general anesthetic. Many IP patients are at an increased risk for VTE at baseline due to underlying comorbidities, including malignancy and chronic hypoxia. Therefore, it is our recommendation that a VTE risk assessment should be performed in all patients in order to develop an appropriate plan of perioperative VTE prophylaxis. The most commonly used tool is the Caprini Score (http://venousdisease.com/dvt-risk-assessment-online/) [42]. Patients with the lowest risk score (0) need only early ambulation during their hospitalization. However, patients with the highest risk scores (≥8) are recommended to have compression boots and prophylactic anticoagulation for 30 days total. Given a lack of consensus guidelines for procedural patients, development of institutional multi-specialty policies can assist in the management of patients at high-risk for VTE, for whom a 30-day prophylactic regimen can be a potentially life-saving intervention.

2.2.6.1 Obstructive Sleep Apnea Screening

It is estimated that 9–24% of the general population have obstructive sleep apnea (OSA). Of these patients, 80% of men and 93% of women with moderate-to-severe OSA are undiagnosed [43]. Patients with OSA have a significantly higher rate of postoperative pulmonary complications, overall complications, mortality, and a longer hLOS [44]. These complications can be reduced by preoperative diagnosis and implementation of positive airway pressure (PAP) therapy. One recent study found that 44% of surveyed patients were willing to postpone elective surgery for diagnosis and management of OSA [45].

The STOP-Bang assessment tool is highly sensitive for OSA. Patients with a positive STOP-Bang Questionnaire identified mild OSA (AHI > 5) in 84% of cases, 93% of moderate OSA (AHI > 15), and 100% of severe OSA cases (AHI > 30) [46, 47]. The specificity of the questionnaire is fairly low (37–56%), and patients deemed high risk for OSA via the STOP-Bang questionnaire should proceed with a formal sleep study for diagnosis.

Reported snoring, observed apnea, tiredness during the daytime, hypertension, BMI > 35 kg/m2, male gender, and increased neck circumference (>41 cm in females and >43 cm in males) are associated with increased OSA risk. Ultimately, all patients with a high risk for OSA should be further assessed with a sleep study. In our clinic, nearly every patient referred for testing has ultimately been diagnosed with sleep apnea, and most of these cases were found to be severe. Sleep studies can now be performed in a patient's own home and interpreted remotely. In our institutional experience, most patients are willing to undergo testing when counselled on the importance of testing and treatment. Untreated sleep apnea worsens the quality of daily living, impacts multiple comorbidities, and shortens life expectancy significantly. In fact, a recent study that compared mortality in patients with treated versus untreated sleep apnea found that those who were compliant with PAP therapy had a 62% reduction in all-cause mortality over 10 years [48].

2.2.6.2 Frailty Assessment

Frailty is a poorly defined high-risk state that portends negative surgical outcomes across all patients presenting for surgical procedures [49]. It has been described as a preexisting pro-inflammatory state characterized by increased levels of cytokines such as IL-6, TNF-alpha, and CRP, as well as hormonal derangements, including elevated cortisol and insulin resistance.

Frail patients have increased rates of mortality (18% compared to baseline of 3%), as well as readmissions, falls, and disability [50]. Frailty can be difficult to study due to the often-present comorbidities that can confound data interpretation.

Two approaches have emerged in the last decade that aim to define and identify frailty in a clinically relevant and feasible fashion. The frailty phenotype (Fried phenotype) [51] is a binary screening model proposed by Fried et al. that includes grip strength, gait speed, physical activity, weight loss, and exhaustion. The Frailty index (FI) is more sensitive in detecting frailty but is burdensome to perform, incorporating 30+ measures [52]. Out of the numerous scoring tools, the FI score, the Fatigue, Resistance, Ambulation, Illness, and Loss of weight (FRAIL) index, the Clinical Frailty Scale (CFS), and the Fried phenotype have the best predictive power for disability and mortality [53].

Regardless of the screening tool utilized, recognizing frail patients in the preanesthetic period and implementing basic interventions has been shown to be a cost-effective way to improve surgical outcomes and reduce hLOS [54]. Compared to the general surgery population, the IP patient population is likely disproportionately frail, and though similar studies have not been performed in IP patients, frailty assessment and optimization are likely beneficial in both the short and long term.

Malnutrition in surgical patients is associated with increased adverse postoperative outcomes, including SSI, hLOS, morbidity, and mortality [32]. In elderly patients, malnutrition is associated with frailty and sarcopenia, both of which are strongly associated with adverse postoperative outcomes. There are dozens of nutritional screening tools to help identify malnourished oncologic, elderly, and hospitalized patients. The Perioperative Nutrition Screening Score (PONS score) was developed specifically for preoperative patients. It takes into account BMI, recent changes in weight, recent decrease in dietary intake, and preoperative albumin level [55].

2.3 Preoperative Optimization of the IP Patient

IP patients often have significant pulmonary disease that must be carefully evaluated during the preanesthetic visit in order to identify opportunities for optimization and tailor a safe anesthetic plan. Next, we discuss optimization and evaluation of these patients; while anesthetic planning will be discussed in later chapters.

2.3.1 Chronic Obstructive Pulmonary Disease

Chronic obstructive pulmonary disease (COPD) has an estimated global prevalence of 10.3% in the adult population [56]. COPD was the third leading cause of death in the United States in 2011 and the cause of an estimated three million annual deaths worldwide in 2024 [56]. The most common cause of COPD is cigarette smoking, and smoking cessation is the most important intervention to improve long-term outcomes in COPD patients. The Global Initiative for Chronic Obstructive Lung Disease (GOLD) 2024 update classifies COPD patients (defined as FEV1/FVC < 0.7) into three groups (ABE) based on symptomatology and exacerbation risk (Table 2.3) and into four categories based on forced expiratory volume in 1 second (FEV1) (Table 2.4) [56].

A thorough history is important to elucidate the severity of symptoms, new or worsening dyspnea, changes in cough or sputum, signs of infection, frequency of acute exacerbations of COPD (ECOPD), and functional capacity. Wheezing on exam is common, while focal findings suggestive of lobar pneumonia may trigger a chest radiograph. An ECOPD increases the risk of pulmonary complications further, and it is recommended for nonurgent procedures to wait at least 6 weeks following their most recent exacerbation. In patients with frequent exacerbations, however, a 6-week

Table 2.3 COPD staging and severity

Stage	FEV1	Severity
GOLD1	FEV1 ≥ 80%	Mild COPD
GOLD2	50% ≤ FEV1 < 80%	Moderate COPD
GOLD3	30% ≤ FEV1 < 50%	Severe COPD
GOLD4	FEV1 < 30%	Very severe COPD

COPD chronic obstructive pulmonary disease, *FEV1* forced expiratory volume in one second

Table 2.4 COPD grouping and treatment [56]

	Symptoms	
Annual exacerbations	Mild mMRC 0–1, CAT <10	Moderate to severe mMRC ≥2, CAT ≥10
0–1 Moderate exacerbation	Group A Bronchodilator Smoking cessation Vaccination	Group B LABA + LAMA Smoking cessation Vaccination Pulmonary rehab
≥2 Moderate exacerbations *and/or* ≥1 hospitalization	Group E LABA + LAMA Consider + ICS if asthma or incr eosinophils Smoking cessation Vaccination Pulmonary rehab	

COPD chronic obstructive pulmonary disease, *mMRC* modified Medical Research Council dyspnea scoring tool, *CAT* COPD Assessment Test, *LABA* long-acting beta agonist, *LAMA* long-acting muscarinic antagonist, *ICS* inhaled corticosteroids window may be difficult to achieve, and it is reasonable to proceed when the patient is otherwise recovered and back to their baseline pulmonary status.

Prophylactic oral steroid administration was thought to reduce ECOPD and pulmonary complications after anesthesia; however, this has been shown to be false and is no longer recommended [57]. Patients on <10 mg/day prednisone having IP procedures do not require stress dosing on the day of their procedure; however, they should continue their oral steroid uninterrupted. Stress dose steroids may be considered in patients on high doses of oral steroids undergoing extensive IP procedures and/or experiencing refractory hypotension under anesthesia [57].

Decreased air movement, accessory muscle use, clubbing of the digits, and/or signs of muscle wasting may be seen on exam and are suggestive of late-stage COPD. While IP procedures are not elective, COPD patients are at an elevated risk of pulmonary complications and should be optimized prior to anesthesia. This includes continuing prescribed pulmonary therapy (medications, oxygen, and/or pulmonary rehab), regular evaluation by pulmonology, adherence with recommended vaccinations, and smoking cessation (discussed below).

Patients with COPD should continue all medications up to and including the day of their procedure. Common medications include short-acting bronchodilators, inhaled corticosteroids, long-acting beta agonists, and muscarinic antagonists [58]. Patients should bring with them on the day of the procedure their short-acting inhalers, portable oxygen, and/or noninvasive positive airway pressure mask and machine.

The primary pulmonology team or primary care provider managing COPD should be made aware of the scheduled procedure and planned general anesthetic. We typically reach out to them to ask if anything further can be done to optimize the patient prior to the procedure. The assessment of a provider with a long-term therapeutic relationship provides valuable insight and information to assess their current state of overall health. COPD is commonly associated with other concomitant morbidities, including frailty, malnutrition, heart failure, hypertension, and diabetes, all of which lead to increased mortality in this population [59]. A comprehensive assessment should therefore include screening and management of coexisting disease.

Patients with very severe COPD (FEV1 < 30%) may present for bronchoscopic lung volume reduction to reduce symptoms and frequency of exacerbations. Specifics of this procedure are discussed in more detail later in the book.

2.3.2 Pulmonary Rehabilitation

Physical activity is essential for all patients, but in patients with chronic pulmonary disease there can be a tendency toward inactivity due to difficulty with dyspnea on exertion. Unfortunately, inactivity worsens long-term outcomes and leads to functional decline. A structured pulmonary rehabilitation program can help improve cardiopulmonary fitness, slow functional decline, reduce symptoms, and decrease the risk of hospitalization with exacerbation [56]. Pulmonary rehabilitation has also been shown to reduce anxiety and depression in COPD patients [60].

A referral to pulmonary rehabilitation should be considered in patients with persistent symptoms of chronic lung disease that interfere with their quality of life. Any patient with an acute ECOPD should be referred to pulmonary rehabilitation, ideally within 3 weeks of onset of symptoms [60]. Other patients who qualify for pulmonary rehabilitation include patients with GOLD II-IV COPD (demonstrated by PFTs) and/or other chronic respiratory disease.

Typical treatment includes sessions three times a week for 6–12 weeks. The six essential components of an American Association of Cardiovascular and Pulmonary Rehabilitation-certified programs include entry assessment and goal setting, education and disease self-management strategies, exercise training and physician conditioning, psychosocial intervention and support, nutritional and pharmacologic intervention, and outcomes assessment [61]. Transportation, time, and costs associated with this commitment can result in decreased participation over time and a reluctance to adhere to treatment recommendations despite the fact that pulmonary rehabilitation programs have been shown to be extremely cost-effective.

There are some data in the preoperative literature that preoperative pulmonary rehabilitation programs can help reduce pulmonary complications in high-risk patients, including those undergoing cardiac or lung-resection surgery. While it is unclear if we can extrapolate these data directly to the IP patient population, the benefits of pulmonary rehab are clear for long-term outcomes. Pulmonary rehab should, therefore, be encouraged and facilitated for IP patients seen in the preanesthesia clinic.

2.3.3 Smoking

Smoking cessation in the preoperative period has been shown to result in higher rates of long-term cessation than in smokers who quit at other times [62]. The majority of patients are motivated to quit, and the preoperative assessment is an opportunity to support cessation. It is well known that smoking results in widespread physiologic detriment. In the preoperative literature, smokers have an increased 30-day mortality and major morbidity, including PPCs, SSIs, ICU admissions, wound complications, neurologic complications, and septic shock [40, 63]. Smoking leads to impaired tissue oxygenation, impaired wound healing, and immunosuppression by neutrophil activity inhibition [64, 65]. Smoking cessation can decrease these effects to near nonsmoker levels. Even brief periods of cessation can be beneficial in reducing wound and pulmonary complications [66].

Given these findings, longer durations of cessation are recommended, with at least 4 weeks of cessation being optimal. Smoking cessation counseling and treatment is an important component of prehabilitation programs where other modifiable patient risk factors can also be addressed [55]. Serum nicotine testing, a sensitive and specific method to verify abstinence from smoking, is typically performed and may therefore improve a patient's chance of smoking cessation compared to traditional self-reporting methods [67].

2.3.4 Pulmonary Hypertension

Pulmonary hypertension (PH) is a pathologic disorder of abnormally elevated blood pressure in the pulmonary arteries. The 6th World Symposium on Pulmonary Hypertension (WSPH) formally defines PH as a mean pulmonary artery pressure (mPAP) ≥20 mmHg measured via right heart catheterization [68]. Increasing use of echocardiography and heightened awareness of PH have increased the overall incidence of diagnosed disease. The prevalence of PH is approximately 1% in the global population, 5% of individuals living at high altitude, and up to 10% of individuals over 65 years of age [69]. The WSPH classifies patients into five groups based on the underlying etiology of disease [68].

Regardless of the type of PH, the most important determining factor for postoperative outcomes is preoperative functional status, classified according to the World Health Organization Functional Classification (WHO-FC) (Table 2.5) [5]. Patients who are asymptomatic with strenuous or regular activity are likely to do well (WHO Group I/II), whereas the mortality of patients with symptoms with mild activity or at rest (WHO groups III/IV) is high [70]. Other worrisome signs in PH patients include recent worsening of symptoms, syncope/pre-syncope with exertion, right ventricular (RV) dilation on cardiac imaging, and signs of RV overload on exam [71].

Pulmonary hypertension is classified into groups based on the etiology of the disease. Patients with pulmonary hypertension from chronic pulmonary disease have group 3 pulmonary hypertension. This is the second most common type of PH. The PERFECT study investigating inhaled Treprostinil in pulmonary hypertension associated with COPD did not show a benefit to inhaled prostaglandins in this population [72]. There are currently no PH-specific therapies for group 3 PH, and the mainstay of treatment is optimization of pulmonary disease.

Management of other groups of PH is beyond the scope of this chapter. But we will briefly summarize salient points. By far, the most common type of PH is group 2, or PH secondary to left heart disease, and approximately 75% of PH patients fall into this category. Diastolic dysfunction, systolic dysfunction, and stenotic or regurgitant valvular disease can all result in elevated pulmonary pressures. Optimization of heart disease is essential for the management of group 2 PH.

Table 2.5 World Health Organization Functional Classification System for patients with pulmonary hypertension [68]

World Health Organization Functional Classification System				
	Class I	Class II	Class III	Class IV
Symptoms with activity	None	Ordinary physical activity causes dyspnea, fatigue, chest pain, or near syncope	Less than ordinary physical activity causes dyspnea, fatigue, chest pain, or near syncope	Dyspnea or fatigue at rest or signs of right heart failure
Functional limitations	None	Slight	Marked limitations	Severe
Comfort level at rest	Comfortable at rest	Comfortable at rest	Comfortable at rest	Symptomatic at rest

Group 1 PH or pulmonary arterial hypertension (PAH) is rare. It is essentially a disease of endothelial hyperproliferation and vasoconstriction [73]. Pharmacotherapy of PAH, therefore, seeks to increase vasodilation and reduce endothelial proliferation through the nitric oxide, endothelin-1, and prostacyclin pathways. These medications should be continued up to and including on the day of surgery.

Group 4 PH chronic thromboembolic pulmonary hypertension (CTEPH) patients are complex and should be treated in a specialized center. These patients should be on lifelong anticoagulation [74]. Riociguat, a medication also used in PAH, reduces mortality in CTEPH patients and should be continued perioperatively. Finally, group 5 PH patients do not fall under any of the above groups and may have systemic comorbid conditions such as connective tissue disorders or rheumatologic disease.

2.3.5 Anemia

Hemorrhage is thankfully rare during IP procedures, and it is typically unnecessary for patients to have blood products available unless severe anemia necessitates a preprocedural transfusion for medical optimization. Patients with pulmonary disease tolerate anemia poorly. If time allows, workup and treatment of mild-to-moderate anemia can be of benefit to patients both periprocedurally and in the long term [75].

Iron deficiency is the most common type of anemia. At our institution, we send iron studies in all anemic patients, including ferritin level and transferrin saturation. The effectiveness of oral iron supplementation is delayed, and it is generally poorly tolerated by patients, so presurgical patients typically qualify for IV iron therapy [75]. Unless there is an obvious reason for the anemia such as recent surgery or menorrhagia, patients should follow up with their primary care provider to determine the etiology of the iron deficiency, with occult gastrointestinal bleeding being the most common cause.

Renal insufficiency is another common cause of preoperative anemia. These patients require treatment with erythropoietin and iron to stimulate their bone marrow to produce additional red blood cells. This may be coordinated with the providers managing the kidney disease. Finally, many IP patients have known or suspected malignancy with a concomitant anemia. In this case, treatment of anemia should be coordinated with their oncology team.

2.3.6 Vaccination

The short-term risks of severe morbidity and mortality are increased in patients with chronic pulmonary disease, who also suffer worsened long-term outcomes following infection secondary to the inflammatory response to infection. Therefore, the lifesaving benefits of vaccination in this population cannot be understated. The Centers for Disease Control (CDC) recommendations for vaccination to SARS-CoV-2 (COVID-19) vary based on strain prevalence but include at least annual vaccination for immunocompetent patients (https://www.cdc.gov/vaccines/hcp/

imz-schedules/adult-age.html) [76]. Additionally, patients with chronic lung disease should have annual influenza, pneumococcal, and respiratory syncytial virus (RSV) vaccines. All patients with COPD should also receive the shingles vaccine series and complete the Tdap vaccination if unvaccinated in adolescence.

2.3.7 Malnutrition

As described above, nutritional status is a modifiable factor of high importance to the perioperative management of surgical patients. It is an independent predictor of surgical outcomes when corrected for other comorbidities and modifiable patient factors [55]. However, there is a paucity of data enabling institutions to develop evidence-based protocols for nutritional optimization. That being said, merely ensuring malnourished patients see a nutritionist preoperatively may improve outcomes. The goal of nutritional prehabilitation is to increase patient nutrient stores that can be accomplished via enteral or parenteral feeding. The use of high protein oral nutritional supplements has been associated with decreased postoperative complications, decreased hLOS, and decreased admission costs [77]. The optimal timeline for intervention is similarly not well studied, and proposed ranges vary widely from 1 week to many months, which may not be feasible in this patient population.

2.3.8 Advance Care Directives

The majority of IP patients are medically complex and elderly. It is now widely recognized that shared decision-making and discussion of advance care directives, code status preferences, and designation of a medical decision-maker is critical in this patient population. [78] Most clinicians possess bias toward life-prolonging treatments, and it is important that we not project these biases onto our patients [79]. An informed discussion of a patient's treatment goals is, therefore, an essential component of patient-focused, geriatric-centered care; however, research has shown that these conversations occur in fewer than half of surgical patients [78–80]. While these studies have been limited to the surgical patient population, it is reasonable to assume that even fewer procedural patients have these discussions with the IP physician, who are predominantly consultants in care and may feel that the discussion is more appropriately handled by the primary care team. More research is clearly warranted in IP patients as they have many comorbid conditions known to be associated with increased risk of undergoing nonbeneficial treatments, including pulmonary disease, long-term oxygen therapy, cancer, and frailty, to name a few [79].

At the very least, all IP patients should have a medical proxy designated and a documented code status discussion prior to consenting for their procedure and anesthesia. A thorough advance care discussion and consultation with palliative care is critical for patients undergoing high-risk procedures, especially if there is consideration for possible postoperative intensive care unit (ICU) admission, prolonged ventilation, or V-V ECMO cannulation.

Cardiopulmonary arrest in the operating room differs from arrest in other situations as it often arises as a consequence of procedural or anesthetic triggers that may be readily treatable and reversible [79]. Therefore, care of the patient with an existing Do-Not-Resuscitate order should entail a detailed discussion of plans for resuscitation during the procedure that align with the patient's stated preferences. These discussions should be facilitated by the physician anesthesiologist and interventional pulmonologist with other members of the care team present when feasible [81]. According to ethical guidelines of the American Society of Anesthesiologists, "Policies automatically suspending DNR orders or other directives that limit treatment prior to procedures involving anesthetic care may not sufficiently address a patient's rights to self-determination in a responsible and ethical manner." [82]

2.4 Summary

The preoperative period is a crucial opportunity to assess and optimize our patients scheduled to undergo interventional pulmonology procedures. Having a thorough, thoughtful, evidence-based process for assessing patients can ensure optimal outcomes, reduce unnecessary case cancellations and delays, shorten hospital stays, and reduce morbidity and mortality. These are all outcomes that patients, pulmonologists, anesthesiologists and hospital leadership are motivated to improve.

References

1. Fischer SP. Development and effectiveness of an anesthesia preoperative evaluation clinic in a teaching hospital. Anesthesiology. 1996;85(1):196–206. https://doi.org/10.1097/00000542-199607000-00025.
2. Ferschl MB, Tung A, Sweitzer B, Huo D, Glick DB. Preoperative clinic visits reduce operating room cancellations and delays. Anesthesiology. 2005;103(4):855–9. https://doi.org/10.1097/00000542-200510000-00025.
3. van Klei WA, Moons KG, Rutten CL, et al. The effect of outpatient preoperative evaluation of hospital inpatients on cancellation of surgery and length of hospital stay. Anesth Analg. 2002;94(3):644–9; table of contents. https://doi.org/10.1097/00000539-200203000-00030.
4. Blitz JD, Kendale SM, Jain SK, Cuff GE, Kim JT, Rosenberg AD. Preoperative evaluation clinic visit is associated with decreased risk of in-hospital postoperative mortality. Anesthesiology. 2016;125(2):280–94. https://doi.org/10.1097/ALN.0000000000001193.
5. Galiè N, Humbert M, Vachiery J-L, et al. 2015 ESC/ERS guidelines for the diagnosis and treatment of pulmonary hypertension. Rev Esp Cardiol (English Ed). 2016;69(2):177. https://doi.org/10.1016/j.rec.2016.01.002.
6. Thompson A, Fleischmann KE, Smilowitz NR, et al. AHA/ACC/ACS/ASNC/HRS/SCA/SCCT/SCMR/SVM guideline for perioperative cardiovascular management for noncardiac surgery: a report of the American College of Cardiology/American Heart Association Joint Committee on Clinical Practice Guidelines. J Am Coll Cardiol. 2024; https://doi.org/10.1016/j.jacc.2024.06.013.
7. Pearson KL, McGuire BE. Anaesthesia for laryngo-tracheal surgery, including tubeless field techniques. BJA Educ. 2017;17(7):242–8. https://doi.org/10.1093/bjaed/mkx004.
8. Crawley SM, Dalton AJ. Predicting the difficult airway. BJA Educ. 2015:15. https://doi.org/10.1093/bjaceaccp/mku047.

9. Mosier J. The physiologically difficult airway and management considerations. Curr Anesthesiol Rep. 2024;14:1–12. https://doi.org/10.1007/s40140-024-00629-w.
10. Nørskov AK, Rosenstock CV, Wetterslev J, Astrup G, Afshari A, Lundstrøm LH. Diagnostic accuracy of anaesthesiologists' prediction of difficult airway management in daily clinical practice: a cohort study of 188 064 patients registered in the Danish Anaesthesia Database. Anaesthesia. 2015;70(3):272–81. https://doi.org/10.1111/anae.12955.
11. Cook TM. Strategies for the prevention of airway complications – a narrative review. Anaesthesia. 2018;73(1):93–111. https://doi.org/10.1111/anae.14123.
12. Law JA, Duggan LV, Asselin M, et al. Canadian Airway Focus Group updated consensus-based recommendations for management of the difficult airway: part 2. Planning and implementing safe management of the patient with an anticipated difficult airway. Can J Anaesth. 2021;68(9):1405–36. Mise à jour des Lignes directrices consensuelles pour la prise en charge des voies aériennes difficiles du Canadian Airway Focus Group : 2(ème) partie. Planification et mise en œuvre d'une prise en charge sécuritaire du patient présentant des voies respiratoires difficiles anticipées. https://doi.org/10.1007/s12630-021-02008-z.
13. Barnwell N, Lenihan M. Anaesthesia for airway stenting. BJA Educ. 2022;22(4):160–6. https://doi.org/10.1016/j.bjae.2021.11.010.
14. Ruetzler K, Bustamante S, Schmidt MT, et al. Video Laryngoscopy vs Direct Laryngoscopy for Endotracheal Intubation in the Operating Room: a cluster randomized clinical trial. JAMA. 2024;331(15):1279–86. https://doi.org/10.1001/jama.2024.0762.
15. Hansel J, Rogers AM, Lewis SR, Cook TM, Smith AF. Videolaryngoscopy versus direct laryngoscopy for adults undergoing tracheal intubation. Cochrane Database Syst Rev. 2022;4(4):Cd011136. https://doi.org/10.1002/14651858.CD011136.pub3.
16. Apfelbaum JL, Hagberg CA, Connis RT, et al. American Society of Anesthesiologists Practice Guidelines for Management of the Difficult Airway. Anesthesiology. 2022;136(1):31–81. https://doi.org/10.1097/aln.0000000000004002.
17. Abdelmalak BB, Doyle DJ. Updates and controversies in anesthesia for advanced interventional pulmonology procedures. Curr Opin Anaesthesiol. 2021;34(4):455–63. https://doi.org/10.1097/aco.0000000000001029.
18. Mahmood K, Frazer-Green L, Gonzalez AV, et al. Management of central airway obstruction: an American College of Chest Physicians Clinical Practice Guideline. Chest. 2024; https://doi.org/10.1016/j.chest.2024.06.3804.
19. Ost DE, Ernst A, Grosu HB, et al. Therapeutic bronchoscopy for malignant central airway obstruction: success rates and impact on dyspnea and quality of life. Chest. 2015;147(5):1282–98. https://doi.org/10.1378/chest.14-1526.
20. Hagberg CA, Artime CA, Aziz MF. Hagberg and Benumof's airway management. 5th ed. Elsevier; 2023: xix, 972 pages.
21. Cook TM, Woodall N, Frerk C. Major complications of airway management in the UK: results of the Fourth National Audit Project of the Royal College of Anaesthetists and the Difficult Airway Society. Part 1: anaesthesia. Br J Anaesth. 2011;106(5):617–31. https://doi.org/10.1093/bja/aer058.
22. Joffe AM, Aziz MF, Posner KL, Duggan LV, Mincer SL, Domino KB. Management of difficult tracheal intubation: a closed claims analysis. Anesthesiology. 2019;131(4):818–29. https://doi.org/10.1097/aln.0000000000002815.
23. Popat M, Mitchell V, Dravid R, Patel A, Swampillai C, Higgs A. Difficult airway society guidelines for the management of tracheal extubation. Anaesthesia. 2012;67(3):318–40. https://doi.org/10.1111/j.1365-2044.2012.07075.x.
24. Malpas G, Hung O, Gilchrist A, et al. The use of extracorporeal membrane oxygenation in the anticipated difficult airway: a case report and systematic review. Can J Anaesth. 2018;65(6):685–97. Recours à l'oxygénation extracorporelle en prévision de la gestion de voies respiratoires difficiles : rapport de cas et étude systématique. https://doi.org/10.1007/s12630-018-1099-x.
25. Kim CW, Kim DH, Son BS, et al. The feasibility of extracorporeal membrane oxygenation in the variant airway problems. Ann Thorac Cardiovasc Surg. 2015;21(6):517–22. https://doi.org/10.5761/atcs.oa.15-00073.

26. Cardarelli MG, Young AJ, Griffith B. Use of extracorporeal membrane oxygenation for adults in cardiac arrest (E-CPR): a meta-analysis of observational studies. Asaio J. 2009;55(6):581–6. https://doi.org/10.1097/MAT.0b013e3181bad907.
27. Colla CH, Morden NE, Sequist TD, Schpero WL, Rosenthal MB. Choosing wisely: prevalence and correlates of low-value health care services in the United States. J Gen Intern Med. 2015;30(2):221–8. https://doi.org/10.1007/s11606-014-3070-z.
28. Cohn SL. Preoperative evaluation for noncardiac surgery. Ann Intern Med. 2016;165(11):Itc81–itc96. https://doi.org/10.7326/aitc201612060.
29. Committee ADAPP. 2. Diagnosis and classification of diabetes: standards of Care in Diabetes—2024. Diabetes Care. 2023;47(Supplement_1):S20–42. https://doi.org/10.2337/dc24-S002.
30. Bang TJ, Chung JH, Walker CM, et al. ACR appropriateness criteria® routine chest imaging. J Am Coll Radiol. 2023;20(5s):S224–33. https://doi.org/10.1016/j.jacr.2023.02.006.
31. Otto CM, Nishimura RA, Bonow RO, et al. 2020 ACC/AHA guideline for the management of patients with valvular heart disease: a report of the American College of Cardiology/American Heart Association Joint Committee on clinical practice guidelines. J Thorac Cardiovasc Surg. 2021;162(2):e183–353. https://doi.org/10.1016/j.jtcvs.2021.04.002.
32. Keeratichananont W, Thanadetsuntorn C, Keeratichananont S. Value of preoperative 6-minute walk test for predicting postoperative pulmonary complications. Ther Adv Respir Dis. 2016;10(1):18–25. https://doi.org/10.1177/1753465815615509.
33. Doherty JU, Daugherty SL, Kort S, et al. ACC/AHA/ASE/ASNC/HFSA/HRS/SCAI/SCCT/SCMR/STS 2024 appropriate use criteria for multimodality imaging in cardiovascular evaluation of patients undergoing nonemergent, noncardiac surgery. J Am Coll Cardiol. 2024; https://doi.org/10.1016/j.jacc.2024.07.022.
34. Herrmann SD, Willis EA, Ainsworth BE, et al. 2024 adult compendium of physical activities: a third update of the energy costs of human activities. J Sport Health Sci. 2024;13(1):6–12. https://doi.org/10.1016/j.jshs.2023.10.010.
35. Hlatky MA, Boineau RE, Higginbotham MB, et al. A brief self-administered questionnaire to determine functional capacity (the Duke Activity Status Index). Am J Cardiol. 1989;64(10):651–4. https://doi.org/10.1016/0002-9149(89)90496-7.
36. Goldman L, Caldera DL, Nussbaum SR, et al. Multifactorial index of cardiac risk in noncardiac surgical procedures. N Engl J Med. 1977;297(16):845–50. https://doi.org/10.1056/nejm197710202971601.
37. Gupta PK, Gupta H, Sundaram A, et al. Development and validation of a risk calculator for prediction of cardiac risk after surgery. Circulation. 2011;124(4):381–7. https://doi.org/10.1161/circulationaha.110.015701.
38. Bilimoria KY, Liu Y, Paruch JL, et al. Development and evaluation of the universal ACS NSQIP surgical risk calculator: a decision aid and informed consent tool for patients and surgeons. J Am Coll Surg. 2013;217(5):833–42.e1–3. https://doi.org/10.1016/j.jamcollsurg.2013.07.385.
39. Liu Y, Cohen ME, Hall BL, Ko CY, Bilimoria KY. Evaluation and enhancement of calibration in the American College of Surgeons NSQIP surgical risk calculator. J Am Coll Surg. 2016;223(2):231–9. https://doi.org/10.1016/j.jamcollsurg.2016.03.040.
40. Chandler D, Mosieri C, Kallurkar A, et al. Perioperative strategies for the reduction of postoperative pulmonary complications. Best Pract Res Clin Anaesthesiol. 2020;34(2):153–66. https://doi.org/10.1016/j.bpa.2020.04.011.
41. Canet J, Gallart L, Gomar C, et al. Prediction of postoperative pulmonary complications in a population-based surgical cohort. Anesthesiology. 2010;113(6):1338–50. https://doi.org/10.1097/ALN.0b013e3181fc6e0a.
42. Caprini JA. Risk assessment as a guide to thrombosis prophylaxis. Curr Opin Pulm Med. 2010;16(5):448–52. https://doi.org/10.1097/MCP.0b013e32833c3d3e.
43. Singh M, Liao P, Kobah S, Wijeysundera DN, Shapiro C, Chung F. Proportion of surgical patients with undiagnosed obstructive sleep apnoea. Br J Anaesth. 2013;110(4):629–36. https://doi.org/10.1093/bja/aes465.
44. Memtsoudis SG, Stundner O, Rasul R, et al. The impact of sleep apnea on postoperative utilization of resources and adverse outcomes. Anesth Analg. 2014;118(2):407–18. https://doi.org/10.1213/ane.0000000000000051.

45. Ho G, Cozowicz C, Wong J, et al. Patient preference survey: are patients willing to delay surgery if obstructive sleep apnea is suspected? BMC Anesthesiol. 2018;18(1):128. https://doi.org/10.1186/s12871-018-0594-5.
46. Chung F, Subramanyam R, Liao P, Sasaki E, Shapiro C, Sun Y. High STOP-Bang score indicates a high probability of obstructive sleep apnoea. Br J Anaesth. 2012;108(5):768–75. https://doi.org/10.1093/bja/aes022.
47. Chung F, Yegneswaran B, Liao P, et al. STOP questionnaire: a tool to screen patients for obstructive sleep apnea. Anesthesiology. 2008;108(5):812–21. https://doi.org/10.1097/ALN.0b013e31816d83e4.
48. Lisan Q, Van Sloten T, Marques Vidal P, Haba Rubio J, Heinzer R, Empana JP. Association of Positive Airway Pressure Prescription with Mortality in Patients with Obesity and Severe Obstructive Sleep Apnea: the Sleep Heart Health Study. JAMA Otolaryngol Head Neck Surg. 2019;145(6):509–15. https://doi.org/10.1001/jamaoto.2019.0281.
49. Richards SJG, Frizelle FA, Geddes JA, Eglinton TW, Hampton MB. Frailty in surgical patients. Int J Color Dis. 2018;33(12):1657–66. https://doi.org/10.1007/s00384-018-3163-y.
50. Aucoin SD, Hao M, Sohi R, et al. Accuracy and feasibility of clinically applied frailty instruments before surgery: a systematic review and meta-analysis. Anesthesiology. 2020;133(1):78–95. https://doi.org/10.1097/aln.0000000000003257.
51. Fried LP, Tangen CM, Walston J, et al. Frailty in older adults: evidence for a phenotype. J Gerontol A Biol Sci Med Sci. 2001;56(3):M146–M56. https://doi.org/10.1093/gerona/56.3.m146.
52. Rockwood K, Song X, MacKnight C, et al. A global clinical measure of fitness and frailty in elderly people. CMAJ. 2005;173(5):489–95. https://doi.org/10.1503/cmaj.050051.
53. Malmstrom TK, Miller DK, Morley JE. A comparison of four frailty models. J Am Geriatr Soc. 2014;62(4):721–6. https://doi.org/10.1111/jgs.12735.
54. Alvarez-Nebreda ML, Bentov N, Urman RD, et al. Recommendations for preoperative management of frailty from the Society for Perioperative Assessment and Quality Improvement (SPAQI). J Clin Anesth. 2018;47:33–42. https://doi.org/10.1016/j.jclinane.2018.02.011.
55. West MA, Wischmeyer PE, Grocott MPW. Prehabilitation and nutritional support to improve perioperative outcomes. Curr Anesthesiol Rep. 2017;7(4):340–9. https://doi.org/10.1007/s40140-017-0245-2.
56. Global Initiative for Chronic Obstructive Lung Disease (GOLD). Global Strategy for the Diagnosis, Management, and Prevention of Chronic Obstructive Pulmonary Disease (2024 Report). Accessed September 2024, https://goldcopd.org/2024-gold-report/.
57. Chen Cardenas SM, Santhanam P, Morris-Wiseman L, Salvatori R, Hamrahian AH. Perioperative evaluation and management of patients on glucocorticoids. J Endocr Soc. 2022;7(2):bvac185. https://doi.org/10.1210/jendso/bvac185.
58. Pfeifer KJ, Selzer A, Whinney CM, et al. Preoperative Management of Gastrointestinal and Pulmonary Medications: Society for Perioperative Assessment and Quality Improvement (SPAQI) consensus statement. Mayo Clin Proc. 2021;96(12):3158–77. https://doi.org/10.1016/j.mayocp.2021.08.008.
59. Miller J, Edwards LD, Agustí A, et al. Comorbidity, systemic inflammation and outcomes in the ECLIPSE cohort. Respir Med. 2013;107(9):1376–84. https://doi.org/10.1016/j.rmed.2013.05.001.
60. Cornelison SD, Pascual RM. Pulmonary rehabilitation in the Management of Chronic Lung Disease. Med Clin North Am. 2019;103(3):577–84. https://doi.org/10.1016/j.mcna.2018.12.015.
61. Ries AL, Bauldoff GS, Carlin BW, et al. Pulmonary rehabilitation: joint ACCP/AACVPR evidence-based clinical practice guidelines. Chest. 2007;131(5 Suppl):4s–42s. https://doi.org/10.1378/chest.06-2418.
62. Shi Y, Warner DO. Surgery as a teachable moment for smoking cessation. Anesthesiology. 2010;112(1):102–7. https://doi.org/10.1097/ALN.0b013e3181c61cf9.
63. Grønkjær M, Eliasen M, Skov-Ettrup LS, et al. Preoperative smoking status and postoperative complications: a systematic review and meta-analysis. Ann Surg. 2014;259(1):52–71. https://doi.org/10.1097/SLA.0b013e3182911913.

64. Sørensen LT, Jørgensen S, Petersen LJ, et al. Acute effects of nicotine and smoking on blood flow, tissue oxygen, and aerobe metabolism of the skin and subcutis. J Surg Res. 2009;152(2):224–30. https://doi.org/10.1016/j.jss.2008.02.066.
65. Allen DB, Maguire JJ, Mahdavian M, et al. Wound hypoxia and acidosis limit neutrophil bacterial killing mechanisms. Arch Surg. 1997;132(9):991–6. https://doi.org/10.1001/archsurg.1997.01430330057009.
66. An D, Ayob F, Rajaleelan W, Chung F, Wong J. Preoperative smoking cessation as part of surgical prehabilitation. Can J Anaesth. 2019;66(4):476–9. https://doi.org/10.1007/s12630-018-01283-7.
67. Hart A, Rainer WG, Taunton MJ, Mabry TM, Berry DJ, Abdel MP. Cotinine testing improves smoking cessation before total joint arthroplasty. J Arthroplast. 2019;34(7s):S148–s151. https://doi.org/10.1016/j.arth.2018.11.039.
68. Humbert M, Kovacs G, Hoeper MM, et al. 2022 ESC/ERS guidelines for the diagnosis and treatment of pulmonary hypertension. Eur Respir J. 2023;61(1). https://doi.org/10.1183/13993003.00879-2022.
69. Hoeper MM, Humbert M, Souza R, et al. A global view of pulmonary hypertension. Lancet Respir Med. 2016;4(4):306–22. https://doi.org/10.1016/s2213-2600(15)00543-3.
70. Rajagopal S, Ruetzler K, Ghadimi K, et al. Evaluation and management of pulmonary hypertension in noncardiac surgery: a Scientific Statement From the American Heart Association. Circulation. 2023;147(17):1317–43. https://doi.org/10.1161/cir.0000000000001136.
71. Maron BA. Revised definition of pulmonary hypertension and approach to management: a clinical primer. J Am Heart Assoc. 2023;12(8). https://doi.org/10.1161/jaha.122.029024.
72. Nathan SD, Argula R, Trivieri MG, et al. Inhaled treprostinil in pulmonary hypertension associated with COPD: PERFECT study results. Eur Respir J. 2024;63(6). https://doi.org/10.1183/13993003.00172-2024.
73. Hassoun PM. Pulmonary arterial hypertension. N Engl J Med. 2021;385(25):2361–76. https://doi.org/10.1056/NEJMra2000348.
74. Elhage Hassan M, Vinales J, Perkins S, Sandesara P, Aggarwal V, Jaber WA. Pathogenesis, diagnosis, and management of chronic thromboembolic pulmonary hypertension. Interv Cardiol Clin. 2023;12(3s):e37–49. https://doi.org/10.1016/j.iccl.2024.04.003.
75. Okocha O, Dand H, Avram MJ, Sweitzer B. An effective and efficient testing protocol for diagnosing iron-deficiency anemia preoperatively. Anesthesiology. 2020;133(1):109–18. https://doi.org/10.1097/aln.0000000000003263.
76. CDC. Centers for Disease Control Adult Immunization Schedule Accessed September 2024, https://www.cdc.gov/vaccines/hcp/imz-schedules/adult-age.html.
77. Accarino JJO, Ramsey A, Samarakoon U, et al. Drug allergy in older adults: a study from the United States Drug Allergy Registry. Ann Allergy Asthma Immunol. 2023;131(5):628–636.e2. https://doi.org/10.1016/j.anai.2023.07.024.
78. Chow WB, Rosenthal RA, Merkow RP, Ko CY, Esnaola NF. Optimal preoperative assessment of the geriatric surgical patient: a best practices guideline from the American College of Surgeons National Surgical Quality Improvement Program and the American Geriatrics Society. J Am Coll Surg. 2012;215(4):453–66. https://doi.org/10.1016/j.jamcollsurg.2012.06.017.
79. Cooper Z, Koritsanszky LA, Cauley CE, et al. Recommendations for best communication practices to facilitate goal-concordant care for seriously ill older patients with emergency surgical conditions. Ann Surg. 2016;263(1):1–6. https://doi.org/10.1097/sla.0000000000001491.
80. Godage S, Rowe K, Hu FY, et al. Preoperative code status discussion workflows: targets for improvement in multidisciplinary pathways. J Pain Symptom Manag. 2023;66(1):e35–43. https://doi.org/10.1016/j.jpainsymman.2023.03.010.
81. Anesthesiologists. ASo. Statement on Ethical Guidelines for the Anesthesia Care of Patients with Do-Not-Resuscitate Orders. Updated October 18, 2023.
82. American Society of Anesthesiologists Statement on Ethical Guidelines for the Anesthesia Care of Patients with Do-Not-Resuscitate (DNR) Orders. Updated October 18, 2023. Accessed September 30, 2024, https://www.asahq.org/standards-and-practice-parameters/statement-on-ethical-guidelines-for-the-anesthesia-care-of-patients-with-do-not-resuscitate-orders.

Anesthesia Techniques for Interventional Pulmonary Procedures

3

Junichi Naganuma

3.1 Introduction

Modern technology and newer techniques in both anesthesiology and interventional pulmonology, a subspecialty of pulmonary medicine, have seen remarkable advancements in recent years. An increasing number of patients with significant comorbidities previously deemed "too sick" for traditional open thoracic surgical procedures are now able to undergo minimally invasive interventional pulmonary procedures with flexible or rigid bronchoscopes. With that, however, comes the added challenges of anesthetists to provide safe and effective anesthetic care to these sicker patients, often in the nonoperating room anesthesia (NORA) setting.

Although there continues to be an ongoing discussion regarding the advantages and disadvantages of proceduralist-administered (or proceduralist-supervised) vs. anesthetist-administered sedation, the benefits of providing at least sedation to all patients undergoing interventional pulmonology procedures were recognized as early as in 2011. The American College of Chest Physicians Consensus Statement on the Use of Topical Anesthesia, Analgesia, and Sedation During Flexible Bronchoscopy in Adult Patients in 2011 concluded that "patients' satisfaction and procedure tolerance are significantly improved with sedation," and that "sedation is suggested in all patients undergoing bronchoscopy unless contraindications exist" [1].

Anesthesia techniques for interventional pulmonary procedures are chosen based on several factors, including patient-related factors, procedure-related factors, and proceduralist-related factors.

J. Naganuma (✉)
Department of Anesthesiology, University of California San Diego, San Diego, CA, USA
e-mail: jnaganuma@health.ucsd.edu

M. Sarkiss (ed.), *Anesthesia for Interventional Pulmonary Procedures*,
https://doi.org/10.1007/978-3-032-12007-6_3

Patient-related factors: patient preference, body habitus, extent of central airway obstruction, comorbidities including significant pulmonary hypertension, uncontrolled gastroesophageal reflux disease (GERD), and uncontrolled diabetes mellitus.

Procedure-related factors: duration, complexity, and need for complete patient immobility.

Proceduralist-related factors: preference for certain types of anesthesia and previous experience.

While it is important to keep these factors in mind when deciding on which type of anesthesia to provide to patients, the anesthetist's options range from topical anesthesia, moderate sedation (or "conscious sedation"), monitored anesthesia care (MAC), regional anesthesia, general anesthesia, or a combination of the above.

When different anesthetic techniques are described for procedures occurring in the nonoperating rooms, such as in interventional pulmonary suites where nurses may be the providers administering sedation, different terms indicating patient sedation levels are used interchangeably, and oftentimes incorrectly. Therefore, before discussing the different anesthesia techniques available for interventional pulmonary procedures, a quick review of terminology related to patient sedation level is necessary.

The American Society of Anesthesiologists (ASA) defines patient sedation level as follows [2] (Fig. 3.1).

Minimal sedation (anxiolysis): A drug-induced state during which patients respond normally to verbal commands. Although cognitive function and physical coordination may be impaired, airway reflexes, and ventilatory and cardiovascular functions are unaffected.

Moderate sedation/analgesia ("conscious sedation"): A drug-induced depression of consciousness during which patients respond purposefully to verbal commands, either alone or accompanied by light tactile stimulation. No interventions are required to maintain a patent airway, and spontaneous ventilation is adequate. Cardiovascular function is usually maintained.

Deep sedation/analgesia: A drug-induced depression of consciousness during which patients cannot be easily aroused but respond purposefully following

	Minimal Sedation Anxiolysis	Moderate Sedation/ Analgesia ("Conscious Sedation")	Deep Sedation/ Analgesia	General Anesthesia
Responsiveness	Normal response to verbal stimulation	Purposeful** response to verbal or tactile stimulation	Purposeful** response following repeated or painful stimulation	Unarousable even with painful stimulus
Airway	Unaffected	No intervention required	Intervention may be required	Intervention often required
Spontaneous Ventilation	Unaffected	Adequate	May be inadequate	Frequently inadequate
Cardiovascular Function	Unaffected	Usually maintained	Usually maintained	May be impaired

Fig. 3.1 ASA statement on continuum of depth of sedation: definition of general anesthesia and levels of sedation/analgesia (https://www.asahq.org/standards-and-practice-parameters/statement-on-continuum-of-depth-of-sedation-definition-of-general-anesthesia-and-levels-of-sedation-analgesia)

repeated or painful stimulation. The ability to independently maintain ventilatory function may be impaired. Patients may require assistance in maintaining a patent airway, and spontaneous ventilation may be inadequate. Cardiovascular function is usually maintained.

General anesthesia: A drug-induced loss of consciousness during which patients are not arousable, even by painful stimulation. The ability to independently maintain ventilatory function is often impaired. Patients often require assistance in maintaining a patent airway, and positive pressure ventilation may be required because of depressed spontaneous ventilation or drug-induced depression of neuromuscular function. Cardiovascular function may be impaired.

It should also be mentioned here that the ASA defines "monitored anesthesia care (MAC)" as "a specific anesthesia service performed by a qualified (trained) anesthesia provider, for a diagnostic or therapeutic procedure. Indications for MAC include, but are not limited to, the nature of the procedure, the patient's clinical condition and/or the need for deeper levels of analgesia and sedation than can be provided by moderate sedation (including potential conversion to a general or regional anesthetic). Monitored Anesthesia Care includes all aspects of anesthesia care—a preprocedure assessment and optimization, intraprocedure care and post-procedure management that is inherently provided by a qualified anesthesia provider as part of the bundled specific service" [3].

3.2 Sedation Strategies and Monitoring

As procedures in interventional pulmonology inevitably involve the airway, patients may be at higher risk of developing airway complications. Procedure- and patient-related factors must be considered when formulating a safe and optimal sedation strategy for any interventional pulmonology procedure.

As mentioned above, the patient's sedation level can vary from awake with no sedation, awake with topical anesthesia, minimal sedation, moderate (or "conscious") sedation, deep sedation, to general anesthesia. It is important to emphasize that because the patient's sedation level lies on a dynamic continuum that can easily fluctuate, providers, whether they are nurses or anesthetists, must be cognizant of this possibility and have the appropriate training to be able to rescue patients accordingly, if needed.

3.2.1 Awake with No Sedation

When the flexible bronchoscopy was first introduced in 1968 by Shigeto Ikeda, bronchoscopies were initially being performed without any sedation [4]. While there were no differences in the complication rates of performing bronchoscopies with or without sedation, the use of sedation led to better patient satisfaction and tolerance for the procedure. This has been supported by the American College of

Chest Physicians' 2011 Consensus Guidelines where it recommended sedation "in all patients undergoing bronchoscopy unless contraindications exist" [1].

3.2.2 Topical Anesthesia

Even today, diagnostic flexible bronchoscopies of very short duration and/or for patients with significant cardiac and/or pulmonary comorbidities who may not tolerate anesthesia can be performed with topical anesthesia alone or in combination with sedation.

Local anesthesia, most commonly 2% lidocaine, can be instilled into the airway to minimize unfavorable reflexes such as the cough or the gag reflex. It should be kept in mind that absorption of a large dose of local anesthetics can result in systemic toxicity. For lidocaine, greater than 8.2 mg/kg instilled in the airway has been reported to possibly result in systemic toxicity [5]. Local anesthetic systemic toxicity progresses from central nervous system (CNS) excitation, seizure, then to CNS depression and possibly death. Nurses and anesthesia providers involved in these interventional pulmonary procedures must be aware of this possibility and understand how to treat this condition.

3.2.3 Moderate Sedation

Typically administered by nonanesthesia providers, the most common regimen includes benzodiazepines and/or opioids. Benzodiazepines are beneficial in providing amnesia and anxiolysis. Of the several benzodiazepines available, midazolam is the most common benzodiazepine administered because of its favorable drug profile: rapid onset, short duration of action, and rapid clearance [6]. Intermittent boluses of 0.5–1 mg iv, taking patient's age, weight, and hepatic/renal dysfunction into consideration, are administered to achieve desired effects. Opioids are not only useful for analgesia, but also suppressing cough reflex [6]. Fentanyl is the most commonly used opioid for these interventional pulmonary procedures with intermittent boluses of 25–50 mcg iv administered to desired effect, again taking patient's age, weight, and hepatic/renal dysfunction into consideration.

3.2.4 General Anesthesia

When general anesthesia is chosen as the anesthetic technique for these interventional pulmonology procedures, total intravenous anesthesia (TIVA) is often used. Inhalational anesthetic gas use is not ideal because bronchoscopes, flexible or rigid, are constantly being moved in and out of the patient's airway. It becomes difficult, if not impossible, to reliably monitor patients' depth of anesthesia, placing them at risk for awareness under general anesthesia especially if muscle relaxation is used.

Additional concerns include polluting the procedure suite with inhalational gas unnecessarily and concomitantly exposing personnel present to these gases.

A common regimen for TIVA at most centers is propofol infusion at rates of 100–200 mcg/kg/min combined with ultra-short-acting opioid remifentanil infusion at rates of 0.1–0.2 mcg/kg/min. Along with this regimen, blood pressure support may be necessary with phenylephrine infusion often at rates 25–80 mcg/min. Other regimens may include ketamine or dexmedetomidine infusions.

3.2.5 Monitoring

Regardless of which sedation strategy is selected, patient should be monitored for the duration of the procedure with American Society of Anesthesiologists (ASA) standard monitors [5].

The five ASA standard monitors include

- Pulse oximetry
- Electrocardiogram (ECG)
- Noninvasive blood pressure (NIBP)
- End-tidal carbon dioxide (EtCO2)
- Temperature

Based on patients' comorbidities, additional monitoring may be necessary. For example, arterial lines may be beneficial for those with significant underlying cardiac and/or pulmonary issues. During the lengthier rigid bronchoscopy procedures utilizing jet ventilation, either manual or automated, where $EtCO_2$ monitoring is unreliable or not possible, serial arterial blood gas analysis may be beneficial in titrating patient's ventilation settings and maintaining acceptable pCO2 throughout the procedure, as unrecognized hypercarbia may lead to CO_2 narcosis, resulting in delayed emergence and/or inability to extubate at the conclusion of the procedure.

While controversies with their use exist, processed electroencephalograms are used routinely at some centers to monitor depth of anesthesia, especially when TIVA is the chosen anesthetic technique. The two most commonly used indices clinically are Medtronic's Bispectral Index (BIS) [7] and Masimo's SedLine [8] Patient State Index (PSi) [9], based on the respective manufacturer's proprietary algorithm.

3.2.5.1 Medtronic's Bispectral Index (BIS)

Based on Medtronic's proprietary algorithm, patient's sedation level is given a numerical value ranging from 0 (deep anesthesia) to 100 (fully awake), with 40–60 as the recommended range when keeping patients under general anesthesia [7].

3.2.5.2 Masimo's SedLine Patient State Index (PSi)

Similar to the Medtronic's BIS, Masimo's SedLine utilizes its own proprietary algorithm and assigns patient's sedation level value ranging from 0 (EEG suppression) to 100 (fully awake). Unlike the BIS, PSi of 25–50 is the recommended range for maintaining patients under general anesthesia [8].

In summary, deciding on which sedation strategy to select requires a thorough understanding of patient's comorbidities combined with the procedure being performed. As such, an effective communication between the proceduralist and the anesthetist is crucial to the successful and safe outcome for the patient.

3.3 Role of Bronchoscopic Techniques in Anesthesia Administration

Bronchoscopic procedures can be grouped into the following three categories: (1) diagnostic flexible bronchoscopic procedures, (2) advanced diagnostic bronchoscopic procedures, and (3) therapeutic bronchoscopic procedures. As procedures with flexible bronchoscope vs. rigid bronchoscope differ in procedural duration and the extent of airway stimulation, anesthesia administration must match the needs of these procedures. A summary of the commonly performed interventional pulmonary procedures and their indications is provided next.

3.3.1 Diagnostic Flexible Bronchoscopy

These procedures may be performed under moderate sedation by nonanesthesia providers or monitored anesthesia care (MAC) by anesthesia providers [6, 10, 11].

- Bronchoalveolar lavage (BAL) is used to analyze alveolar contents and diagnose infections, eosinophilic pneumonia, etc. A total of 100–240 ml of sterile normal saline is instilled into the airway [4].
- Transbronchial lung biopsy (TBLB) is used to sample lung parenchyma in pulmonary diseases, including granulomatous diseases, eosinophilic pneumonia, and infections.
- Transbronchial needle aspiration (TBNA) is the sampling of mediastinal and/or hilar lymphadenopathy through the bronchial or the tracheal wall.
- Bronchial brushings: Bronchial brushings are used in obtaining microbiological and cytological samples of endobronchial lesions and tumors.

3.3.2 Advanced Diagnostic Bronchoscopy

These procedures can be performed with monitored anesthesia care (MAC) or with general anesthesia placing the supraglottic airway, that is, LMA [6, 10, 11].

- Endobronchial ultrasound (EBUS)-TBNA allows needle aspiration biopsies to be taken under real-time ultrasound guidance of the EBUS bronchoscope.

- Radial probe endobronchial ultrasound (RP-EBUS) provides a circumferential radial ultrasound image and is useful in identifying peripheral lung lesions [12].
- Electromagnetic navigational bronchoscopy (ENB) system reconstructs CT scans into 3-D imaging and is used to biopsy peripheral lesions beyond the reach of the bronchoscope.
- Ultrathin bronchoscopy is able to be advanced more distally for peripheral lesions where conventional bronchoscopes could not reach.
- Transbronchial lung cryobiopsy (TBLC) utilizes cryoprobes to obtain lung tissue samples and has been reported to be more advantages than TBLB.

3.3.3 Therapeutic Bronchoscopy

These procedures typically require general anesthesia with muscle relaxation, so an ETT or a rigid bronchoscope is utilized [6, 11].

- Laser bronchoscopy is used to coagulate and vaporize the endobronchial lesion.
- Similar to laser, electrocautery can be used to coagulate and vaporize endobronchial lesions.
- Argon plasma coagulation (APC) is a noncontact type of electrocautery. Similar to the argon beam coagulator used during surgery, it is especially useful in treating bleeding lesions.
- Cryotherapy applies cycles of freezing and thawing to tumors and lesions, ultimately resulting in tissue necrosis.
- Photodynamic therapy is where a photosensitizer substance is administered into the targeted tissue or tumor and is subsequently activated with laser of a certain wavelength and results in tissue necrosis.
- Airway stent placement: Metallic or silicone stents can be deployed into the airway to ameliorate airway stenosis.

In summary, because of the wide variation in procedure times and the extent of airway stimulation during these interventional pulmonology procedures, bronchoscopic technique for a given procedure will determine the anesthesia technique to be selected to meet the needs of the procedure, the proceduralist, and the safety of the patient. It is generally possible to perform procedures involving the flexible bronchoscope under "moderate sedation" or monitored anesthesia care, but those utilizing the right bronchoscope will require general anesthesia.

3.4 Medications Used

Interventional pulmonary procedures are unique in that anesthetists must often share patient's airway with the proceduralist when administering general anesthesia for these procedures. Although the use of inhalational anesthetics such as sevoflurane is certainly possible, most anesthetists would agree that total intravenous anesthesia (TIVA) may be the better choice. This is especially true for the advanced therapeutic procedures mentioned above where procedures are more complex, and therefore lengthier, and complete patient immobility with muscle relaxation is necessary. Moreover, the use of inhalational anesthetics during therapeutic procedures with rigid bronchoscopes is not ideal, given the inevitable leak around the bronchoscope leading to unreliable delivery of anesthetic agent to the patient (and possibly increasing the likelihood of "awareness under general anesthesia") and the unwanted exposure of inhalational anesthetics to the care team present in the procedural suite or the contamination of the working environment with inhalational anesthetics.

Propofol: The most commonly used intravenous hypnotic agent when TIVA is selected as the anesthetic choice and is often administered at doses of 100–200 mcg/kg/min. While cardiopulmonary side effects such as hypotension and respiratory depression are possible, they can easily be treated by qualified anesthetists.

Remifentanil: An ultra-short-acting opioid with rapid onset time and rapid elimination via plasma esterase by Hoffmann degradation, making it an ideal analgesic adjunct when used as part of TIVA at doses of 0.1–0.2 mcg/kg/min with propofol infusion.

Dexmedetomidine: A selective alpha-2 agonist sedative that maintain spontaneous ventilation in patients. Because of its longer onset of action and duration of action compared to propofol and remifentanil mentioned above, it may not be an ideal choice for short procedures such as diagnostic bronchoscopy but may be beneficial as an adjunct to propofol and remifentanil for longer procedures [13].

Ketamine: An N-methyl D-aspartate receptor antagonist and partial agonist at opioid mu-receptors with anesthetic and analgesic properties that maintains spontaneous ventilation. Although increased salivation is an unfavorable side effect for pulmonary procedures, ketamine's bronchodilatory effect and stable cardiovascular profile are ideal properties when using this medication for patients with severe cardiopulmonary comorbidities [14, 15].

3.5 Airway Choice for General Anesthesia with Flexible Bronchoscopy

When general anesthesia is selected as the anesthetic technique for procedures with flexible bronchoscopy, the airway device can either be a laryngeal mask airway (LMA) or an endotracheal tube (ETT), and its selection depends on patient-related and/or procedure-related factors.

Factors that favor LMA placement: A full view of the glottic structures not possible with ETT is necessary; access to higher station cervical and/or paratracheal lymph nodes is required; patient has subglottic stenosis.

Factors that favor ETT placement: Patient-related factors such as morbid obesity, large hiatal hernia, uncontrolled gastroesophageal reflux disease, significant pulmonary hypertension, severe obstructive sleep apnea (OSA), and uncontrolled diabetes mellitus; procedure-related factors such as need for complete muscle relaxation.

3.5.1 Laryngeal Mask Airway (LMA)

If an LMA selected as the airway device, oftentimes for procedures with the flexible bronchoscope, the vocal cords are often sprayed with topical local anesthetics before the bronchoscope is advanced past the vocal cords to avoid coughing and even laryngospasm [16]. With LMAs, peak airway pressure should be kept at less than 20 cm H_2O, to minimize leak around the LMA and gastric distention [13].

3.5.2 Endotracheal Tube (ETT)

If an ETT is selected to secure the airway, the anesthetist and the proceduralist must consider the size, more specifically the inner diameter, of the ETT such that it will accommodate the bronchoscope to be used and still be able to effectively ventilate around the bronchoscope. Most centers would place at least an 8.0 mm ETT for flexible bronchoscope procedures, but some bronchoscopes would require a larger ETT such as an 8.5 mm or even 9.0 mm [17].

3.6 Airway Choice for General Anesthesia with Rigid Bronchoscopy

Because the rigid bronchoscope is essentially a straight metal tube with a beveled distal end that goes into the trachea from the patient's mouth, rigid bronchoscopy usually requires general anesthesia. Since procedures involving rigid bronchoscopes are typically more complex, cases tend to be longer in duration, and because ventilation is paused frequently, they are often performed with TIVA as the anesthetic technique. To add to this complexity, different modes of ventilation must be considered provide optimal condition for the proceduralist, while keeping safety of the patient in mind.

3.6.1 Modes of Ventilation

3.6.1.1 Apneic Oxygenation

This ventilation approach was the original ventilation method for rigid bronchoscopy and is no longer in routine use. With apneic oxygenation, after patients are preoxygenated with 100% FiO2, ventilation is paused while the proceduralist performs the procedure. When the patient's SpO2 drops, the procedure is suspended, bronchoscope is removed, and patient is oxygenated until oxygenation improves.

The proceduralist is then allowed to reinsert the bronchoscope and the procedure resumes [6].

3.6.1.2 Spontaneous-Assisted Ventilation

Under TIVA, patient maintains spontaneous breathing. Anesthesia circuit is attached to the bronchoscope, and the anesthetist supports patient ventilation via anesthesia bag as needed [6].

3.6.1.3 Controlled Mechanical Ventilation

Similar to the "spontaneous-assisted ventilation" above, the anesthesia circuit is attached to the bronchoscope and mechanical ventilation is provided via the anesthesia machine.

3.6.1.4 Jet Ventilation (Manual or Automatic, High or Low Frequency)

The most common ventilation mode used for rigid bronchoscopy. Jet ventilation can be delivered manually or mechanically as high-frequency jet ventilation (120–600 respirations/min) or low-frequency jet ventilation (10–30 respirations/min) [6]. The manual jet ventilator is commonly referred to as the Sanders jet ventilator, named after its inventor Douglas Sanders [18] (Fig. 3.2). Acutronic monsoon jet ventilator is frequently used at most centers when automatic jet ventilation is needed [19] (Fig. 3.3).

3.6.2 Strategies for Effective Ventilation

Even with the newer bronchoscopic-guided technology, diagnostic yield is usually limited by "computed tomography (CT)-to-body divergence," a "mismatch between the preprocedure CT-based virtual map used to plan the navigation route to the lung

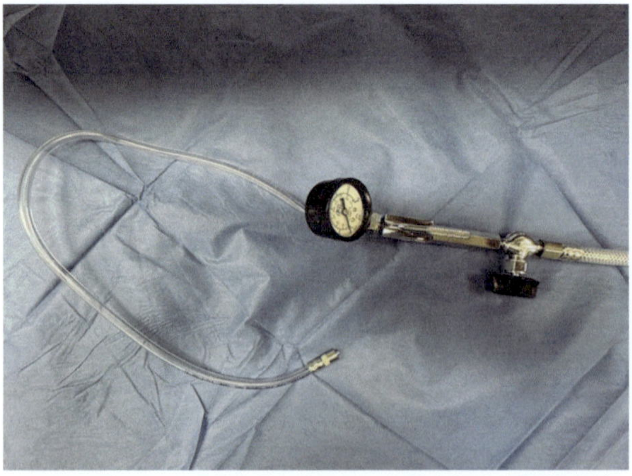

Fig. 3.2 Sanders jet ventilator

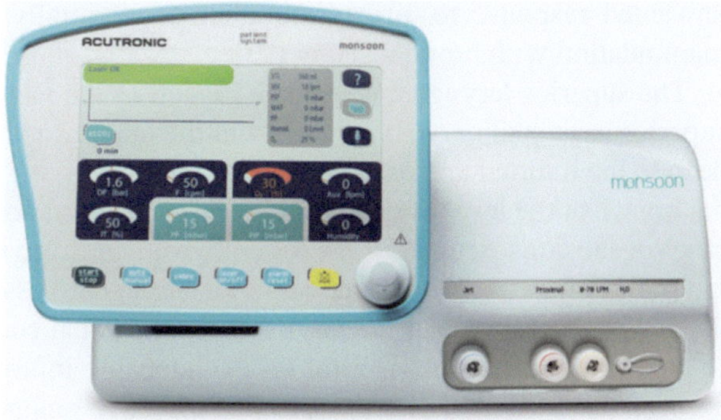

Fig. 3.3 Acutronic's monsoon jet ventilator. (https://www.susquemicro.com/ventilation/monsoon-III-jet-ventilator)

lesion and the actual dynamic lung anatomy during bronchoscopy." Aside from bronchoscopy-related factors that are beyond the anesthesia team's control, addressing anesthesia-related factors such as anesthesia-induced atelectasis could lessen CT-to-body divergence and can subsequently contribute to a better diagnostic yield [20].

Several trials have since addressed the issue of reducing the incidence of atelectasis during bronchoscopy under general anesthesia.

The Ventilatory Strategy to Prevent Atelectasis (VESPA) trial in 2022 compared standard ventilation (LMA, 100% FiO2, zero-positive end-expiratory pressure, PEEP) with VESPA ventilation (ETT followed by a recruitment maneuver, FiO2 titration to <100%, and PEEP of 8–10 cm H2O). The trial showed that this specialized ventilation protocol reduced the incidence of atelectasis with statistical significance [21].

In summary, interventional pulmonary procedures pose unique challenges to anesthetists as we must share the airway with the proceduralists. While topical anesthesia, sedation, or regional anesthesia can be chosen based on factors related to patients, procedure, or proceduralists, general anesthesia is usually selected for advanced diagnostic or advanced therapeutic procedures [22].

3.7 Regional Anesthesia for Pulmonary Interventions

Regional anesthesia, especially ultrasound-guided nerve blocks, has been gaining wider acceptance for various procedures, including interventional pulmonary procedures, as the primary anesthetic or as an adjunct anesthetic in combination with other anesthetic techniques.

3.7.1 Upper Airway Blocks

While not routinely performed for interventional pulmonary procedures, superior laryngeal nerve block (SLNB) can be beneficial as it blunts the cough reflex, an unwanted response to airway stimulation potentially exacerbated during airway manipulation with bronchoscopy [23].

The superior laryngeal nerve is a branch of the vagus nerve in the neck. As the superior laryngeal nerve branches from the main trunk of the vagus nerve, it passes deep to the internal and external carotid arteries, giving off an internal and an external branch at the level of the hyoid bone. The external branch innervates the inferior pharyngeal constrictor and the cricothyroid muscle, while sensory fibers of the internal branch travel with the superior laryngeal vessels as a bundle through the thyrohyoid membrane to the larynx above the vocal cords.

With the injection of 1–2 ml of 2% lidocaine inferior and lateral to the greater horn of the hyoid, SLNB can provide effective analgesia for 60–180 min, while local spraying of lidocaine along the airway mucosa may provide incomplete analgesia for only 8–14 min.

The role of SLNB in awake intubation has been studied previously, and studies have shown that SLNB decreases the time to intubation and improves patient satisfaction. SLNB's usefulness in awake intubation can perhaps be applied as well to bronchoscopic procedures in patients with severe comorbidities who may not tolerate general anesthesia or even sedation [24, 25].

Of the several nerve blocks available in the neck region, SLNB is the most common nerve block to be utilized for bronchoscopic procedures as it provides anesthesia to the larynx above the vocal cords, for example, the epiglottis, aryepiglottic folds, and laryngeal structures to the false cords.

The following upper airway nerve blocks may also be performed in conjunction with SLNB [26, 27]:

Glossopharyngeal nerve block: Provides oropharyngeal anesthesia and attenuates the gag reflex.

Recurrent laryngeal nerve block (trans laryngeal block): provides anesthesia to infraglottic larynx and trachea below the cords and attenuates bronchospasm.

3.7.2 Regional Anesthesia Techniques for Chest Wall Procedures

For procedures involving the chest wall such as pleuroscopy, pleurodesis, adhesiolysis, and pleural decortication, the following chest wall blocks can be performed: [12]

Paravertebral block (PVB): blocks segmental spinal and sympathetic nerves.

Erector spinae plane block (ESPB): blocks dorsal and ventral rami of spinal nerves.

Serratus anterior plane block (SAPB)/interpectoral block (PEC I)/pectoserratus block (PEC II): blocks thoracodorsal nerve, long thoracic nerve, upper and lower subscapular nerve, and lateral cutaneous branch of intercostal nerve.

Intercostal nerve block (ICNB): blocks ventral rami of thoracic nerves.

In summary, regional anesthesia has gained popularity in recent years and its application continues to grow. For interventional pulmonary procedures involving the airway, attenuation of the cough reflex is important. Because superior laryngeal nerve block effectively minimizes the cough reflex, it may be useful as an adjunct, or as the primary anesthetic in patients with significant cardiopulmonary comorbidities who may not tolerate general anesthesia or even sedation.

References

1. Wahidi MM, Jain P, Jantz M, Lee P, Mackensen GB, Barbour SY, et al. American College of Chest Physicians consensus statement on the use of topical anesthesia, analgesia, and sedation during flexible bronchoscopy in adult patients. Chest. 2011;140(5):1342–50.
2. https://www.asahq.org/standards-and-practice-parameters/statement-on-continuum-of-depth-of-sedation-definition-of-general-anesthesia-and-levels-of-sedation-analgesia.
3. https://www.asahq.org/standards-and-practice-parameters/statement-on-distinguishing-monitored-anesthesia-care-from-moderate-sedation-analgesia.
4. Ikeda S, Yanai N, Ishikawa S. Flexible bronchofiberscope. Keio J Med. 1968;17(1):1–16.
5. https://www.asahq.org/standards-and-practice-parameters/standards-for-basic-anesthetic-monitoring.
6. de Lima A, Kheir F, Majid A, Pawlowski J. Anesthesia for interventional pulmonology procedures: a review of advanced diagnostic and therapeutic bronchoscopy. Can J Anaesth. 2018;65(7):822–36.
7. https://www.medtronic.com/en-us/healthcare-professionals/products/patient-monitoring/brain-monitoring/brain-channel-monitoring/bis-monitoring-system.html.
8. https://www.masimo.com/products/continuous/root/root-sedline/.
9. https://www.medtronic.com/content/dam/medtronic-wide/public/united-states/products/patient-monitoring/bis-monitor-perioperative-brain-monitoring-part1-white-paper.pdf.
10. Galway U, Zura A, Khanna S, Wang M, Turan A, Ruetzler K. Anesthetic considerations for bronchoscopic procedures: a narrative review based on the Cleveland Clinic experience. J Thorac Dis. 2019;11(7):3156–70.
11. Díaz-Jimenez JaR A, editor. Interventions in pulmonary medicine; 2023.
12. Sikachi RR, Chaddha U, Agrawal A. Anesthetic considerations for medical pleuroscopy. Respir Med. 2023;213:107225.
13. Goudra BG, Singh PM, Borle A, Farid N, Harris K. Anesthesia for advanced bronchoscopic procedures: state-of-the-art review. Lung. 2015;193(4):453–65.
14. Apostolos F, Nikolaos Z, Charalampos M, Kyriakos K, Sotirios F, Gregorios V. Dexmedetomidine-ketamine combination versus fentanyl-midazolam for patient sedation during flexible bronchoscopy: a prospective, single-blind, randomized controlled trial. BMC Pulm Med. 2024;24(1):301.
15. Jose RJ, Shaefi S, Navani N. Sedation for flexible bronchoscopy: current and emerging evidence. Eur Respir Rev. 2013;22(128):106–16.
16. Abdelmalak BB, Doyle DJ. Updates and controversies in anesthesia for advanced interventional pulmonology procedures. Curr Opin Anaesthesiol. 2021;34(4):455–63.
17. Sarkiss M. Anesthesia for interventional bronchoscopic procedures. In: Díaz-Jimenez JRA, editor. Interventions in pulmonary medicine; 2023.
18. Sanders RD. Two ventilating attachments for bronchoscopes. Del Med J. 39(170):92.
19. https://www.susquemicro.com/ventilation/monsoon-III-jet-ventilator.

20. Pritchett MA, Lau K, Skibo S, Phillips KA, Bhadra K. Anesthesia considerations to reduce motion and atelectasis during advanced guided bronchoscopy. BMC Pulm Med. 2021;21(1):240.
21. Salahuddin M, Sarkiss M, Sagar AS, Vlahos I, Chang CH, Shah A, et al. Ventilatory strategy to prevent atelectasis during bronchoscopy under general anesthesia: a multicenter randomized controlled trial (Ventilatory Strategy to Prevent Atelectasis -VESPA- Trial). Chest. 2022;162(6):1393–401.
22. Frye L. Anesthesia considerations for advanced bronchoscopy: a narrative review. AME Med J. 2024;9(34)
23. Camara RGC. Anatomy of the Vagus nerve, nerves and nerve injuries. Academic Press; 2015. p. 385–97.
24. Okada TYM, Matsushita T, Ishida Y, Furukawa K, Murozono M. Anesthetic management of airway stent placement by rigid bronchoscopy with superior laryngeal nerve block while preserving spontaneous breathing: a case report. Clin Case Rep. 2023;19(11):e8232.
25. Liao YC, Wu WC, Hsieh MH, Chang CC, Tsai HC. Ultrasound-guided superior laryngeal nerve block assists in anesthesia for bronchoscopic surgical procedure: a case report of anesthesia for rigid bronchoscopy. Medicine (Baltimore). 2020;99(27):e20916.
26. Hua Y, Huang Q, Chen G, Zhu T. Comparison of modified anterior and traditional posterior accesses for ultrasound-guided superior laryngeal nerve block in awake endotracheal intubation: study protocol for a randomised non-inferiority clinical trial. BMJ Open. 2023;13(2):e068779.
27. Amri P, Nikbakhsh N, Modaress SR, Nosrati R. Upper airway nerve block for rigid bronchoscopy in the patients with tracheal stenosis: a case serie. Anesth Pain Med. 2020;10(4):e99796.

Rigid Bronchoscopy and Bronchial Interventions

4

Layal Abou Daher, Carlos E. Guerra-Londono, and Labib Gilles Debiane

4.1 Introduction

Interventional pulmonology has grown in both numbers and complexity in recent years [1, 2]. With the perpetual introduction of new technology into this field, interventional pulmonologists can conduct a wide array of procedures ranging from basic diagnostic to advanced complex therapeutic procedures. Such interventions pose a challenge to the anesthesiologist as they often require shared access to the airway, adequate degree of muscle relaxation, and an optimization of oxygenation and ventilation [3]. Therefore, anesthesiologists must acquaint themselves with the unique nuances of the "interventional pulmonary suite." Despite the advancements in flexible bronchoscopy, rigid bronchoscopy has proven itself to stand the test of time and remains the therapeutic instrument of choice for the management of complex airway diseases [4]. This chapter provides insight into the anesthesia considerations for rigid bronchoscopy focusing on pre-procedural evaluation, scope of use, and special anesthetic considerations in particular situations.

4.1.1 Background

As early as the fourth century BC, Hippocrates suggested the introduction of a pipe into the larynx to relieve suffocation. Later in the 1750s, Desault suggested nasotracheal intubation as a treatment for suffocation and foreign body aspiration [4]. Dr.

L. A. Daher · C. E. Guerra-Londono
Department of Anesthesiology, Pain Management, & Perioperative Medicine, Henry Ford Hospital, Detroit, MI, USA
e-mail: laboud1@hfhs.org; cguerra1@hfhs.org

L. G. Debiane (✉)
Henry Ford Hospital, Detroit, MI, USA
e-mail: ldebian1@hfhs.org

M. Sarkiss (ed.), *Anesthesia for Interventional Pulmonary Procedures*,
https://doi.org/10.1007/978-3-032-12007-6_4

Gustav Killian, a German laryngologist, performed the first rigid bronchoscopy in 1876 [5], whereby he successfully removed a foreign body from the right main stem bronchus using an esophagoscope [6]. Later in 1904, the modern-day rigid bronchoscope with distal illumination was developed by Dr. Chevalier Jackson, an American otolaryngologist [7]. Since then, advances continued in 1954 in England, where Hopkins developed a rod-lens telescope system that refined the lighting and imaging, thus enhancing the access to the airways [8]. Karl Storz adopted this technology as a cold light illumination source for his rigid bronchoscopes in 1963 [8].

A rigid bronchoscope is a hollow metal tube of varying diameter size with a beveled distal end that is used to perform complex endobronchial interventions for airway recanalization, thermal ablation, and control of bleeding (Fig. 4.1) [1, 3]. What makes rigid bronchoscopy unique is that it provides the proceduralist the ability to conduct advanced endobronchial interventions while providing ventilation and oxygenation through the same airway access [1]. The use of rigid bronchoscopy is a defining skill for interventional pulmonologists [8].

Rigid bronchoscopy is most often performed in the operating room [3]. Nevertheless, the increasing caseload and proliferation of advanced rigid bronchoscopy procedures have seen it performed in dedicated suites in many tertiary centers [9]. These suites are functionally hybrid operating rooms, suitable for diagnostic and advanced therapeutic interventions that align with current state-of-the-art procedures [9].

The improvement in anesthetic techniques has been equally fundamental to the practice of bronchoscopy [7]. Cocaine was the first local anesthetic introduced by Jellinek in 1884 that allowed Killian to perform his procedures before the development of general anesthesia. It was soon discovered local anesthetics were limited by their inability to reduce patient's anxiety or provide immobility [10]. As a result, mild and moderate procedural sedation started to stir more interest. In contrast to flexible bronchoscopy that can successfully be performed under topical anesthesia and moderate sedation, rigid bronchoscopy more often than not requires general anesthesia [9]. Our reasoning behind this is that conscious sedation does not always guarantee optimal conditions and increases the risk of hypoxemia and loss of airway patency in prolonged cases, diverting the attention of the proceduralist [10]. Finally, regional anesthesia via a superior laryngeal block has also been described but is rarely used [11, 12].

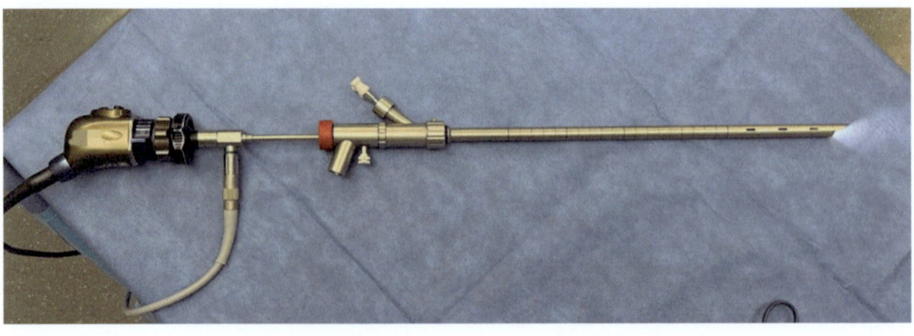

Fig. 4.1 Rigid bronchoscope with light source

4.2 Indications and Contraindications

The principal indications and contraindications for rigid bronchoscopy are summarized in Table 4.1. While indications are easy to accept, most contraindications are relative because rigid bronchoscopy is often a life-saving procedure, forcing clinicians to balance risks and benefits constantly [8]. Due to the need for cervical spine extension during bronchoscope placement, cervical spine instability is the most important absolute contraindication. For others, the expert opinion is mixed. Examples of that are uncontrolled coagulopathy, extreme ventilatory or oxygenation demands, and a tracheal obstruction with a novice operator [4, 8, 13]. Distinction may be based on the severity of coagulopathy, hypoxemia, hemodynamic instability, and urgency of the patient's condition [4, 8]. Finally, the issue of a full stomach (e.g., intestinal obstruction, gastroparesis) must be considered as the airway is not protected from aspiration.

Table 4.1 Indications and contraindications to rigid bronchoscopy

Indications		Contraindications	
Diagnostic	Therapeutic	Absolute	Relative
High-risk endobronchial and transbronchial biopsy (e.g., transbronchial lung cryo-biopsy, biopsy of endobronchial lesions with high bleeding risk)	Central airway obstruction (malignant and nonmalignant): Mechanical tissue debulking Balloon bronchoplasty Rigid dilation Stent placement (particularly silicone Y stents)	Cervical spine instability	Severe coagulopathy
Deeper and larger endobronchial biopsy specimen	Use of thermal ablative techniques (e.g. electrocautery, laser, argon plasma coagulation)		High ventilation/ oxygenation requirements
	Massive hemoptysis		Recent cardiac or neurologic compromise
	Foreign body removal		Presence of aortic aneurysm
			Neuromuscular conditions worsened by paralytics
			Hemodynamic instability
			Limited mouth opening
			Facial fractures

Diaz-Mendoza et al. [8]

4.3 Preoperative Planning

Anesthetic planning begins with preoperative patient evaluation, airway assessment, and optimization, which may be limited in emergencies [9]. Routine premedication is generally not recommended as it may cause acute-on-chronic respiratory failure [9]. If done, supplemental oxygen is strongly advised. Administering antisialogogues such as glycopyrrolate or atropine is also not routinely necessary [14, 15].

Patients presenting for interventional pulmonology procedures are generally classified as American Society of Anesthesiology Physical Status (ASA PS) 3 or greater because of their complex, high-risk, airway disease [16]. Preoperative evaluation includes a history and physical exam focused on common comorbidities that reduce the cardiopulmonary reserve from anesthetic induction or sedation [2]. Ultimately, oxygenation and ventilation will depend on the proper manual placement of the rigid bronchoscope. Detecting conditions that accelerate desaturation or hemodynamic decompensation, impede manual bag-valve-mask ventilation, or suggest a difficult bronchoscope placement is therefore critical. Examples include chronic obstructive pulmonary disease (COPD), obesity, obstructive sleep apnea (OSA), congestive heart failure, and pulmonary hypertension. Overall, the aim is to detect patients whose respiratory function is more likely to be adversely affected by anesthesia and mitigate postoperative pulmonary complications [17]. Whenever possible, specific intra or postprocedural needs can help determine whether the procedure is appropriate for the planned suite or hospital. Preprocedural imaging (e.g., computed tomography) can inform about the nature, location, and size of the lesion in patients with intraluminal airway obstruction. Despite the advanced disease, most patients undergoing rigid bronchoscopy do not require preoperative pulmonary function testing as it will not modify the management. Routine pulmonary function testing is only indicated for bronchoscopic lung volume reduction (BLVR).

Clinical assessment includes recognizing signs and symptoms of a compromised airway (shortness of breath, use of accessory muscles, orthopnea, tachypnea, wheezing, stridor, hoarseness, and bleeding) [9]. The presence of stridor before the procedure must alert the likelihood of narrowing of the upper airway [2]. Some patients may be on home oxygen or may need bronchodilators preoperatively. Furthermore, evaluating functional capacity, respiratory rate, and respiratory pattern aids in the clinical judgment of respiratory compromise [16]. A discussion with the pulmonologist is helpful for better understanding and communication on the exact intraoperative plan.

Data suggest that age (greater than 60 years), preexisting lung disease, smoking, spirometry (FEV1 < 1 L), and duration of anesthesia (>3 h) are independent predictors of worsening pulmonary outcomes postoperatively [18]. Finally, patients with a history of cervical spine fusion, instability, rheumatoid arthritis, as well as radiation to the neck can be at an increased risk of atlantoaxial subluxation or worsening neurologic symptoms [8].

4.3.1 Operating Room Set-Up

The interventional pulmonology team ensures the presence of the required bronchoscopy equipment aided by various light sources, telescopes, and accessory instruments such as laser fibers, cryotherapy, electrocautery probes, balloon dilators, and stents and retrieval forceps [19]. Since 2002, the European Respiratory Society and the American Thoracic Society (ERS/ATS) recommended that the design of the bronchoscopy suite should account for the presence of proper anesthesia equipment (Fig. 4.2) [19].

Typical equipment includes standard ASA monitoring equipment (pulse oximetry, heart rate, five-lead electrocardiogram, blood pressure, and temperature), rescue medications, and various airway equipment such as nasal airway, oral airway, laryngeal mask airway (LMA), endotracheal tube (ETT), intubating stylets, self-inflating bag-valve-mask, suction, and a video laryngoscope. An ETT should be available in a wide range of sizes, as small as 5.0 mm for cases of tracheal stenosis and as large as 9.0–10.0 mm for cases of massive hemoptysis. In addition,

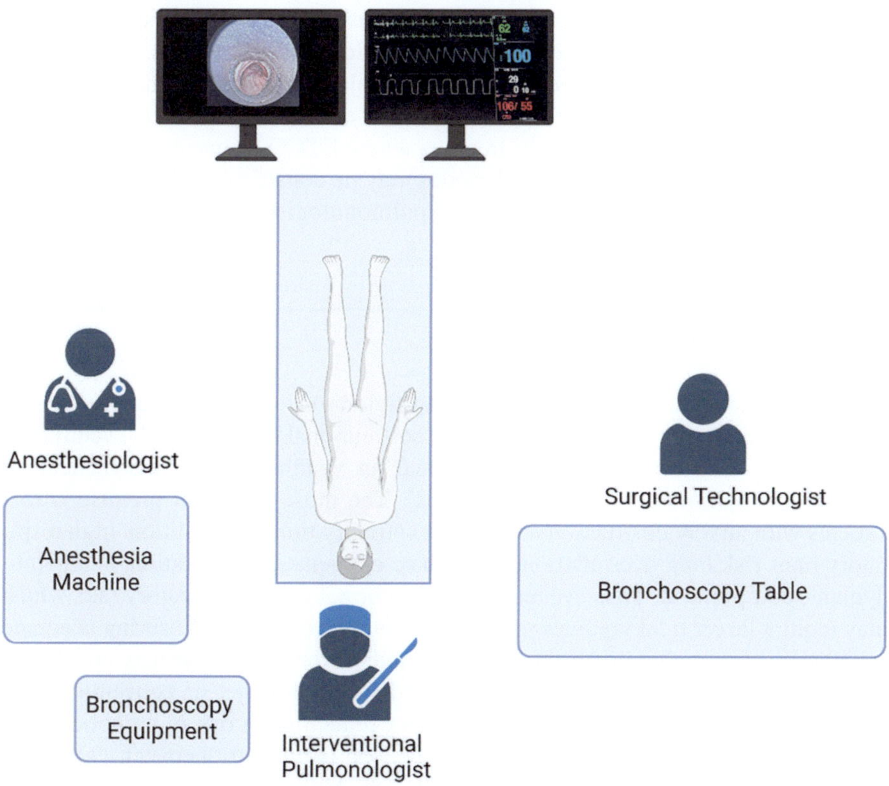

Fig. 4.2 Interventional pulmonology suite design (example)

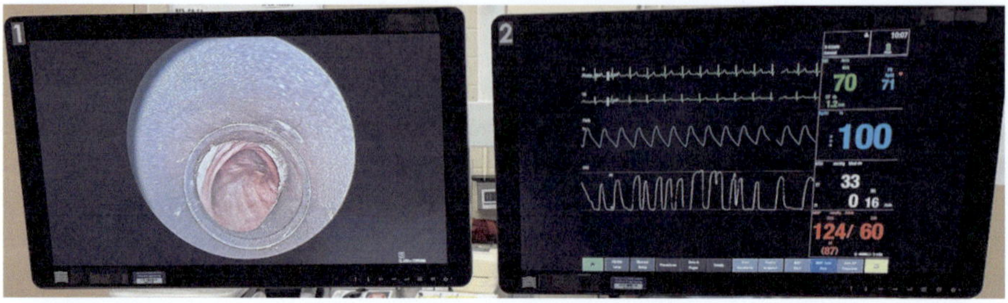

Fig. 4.3 Shared display of bronchoscopy and clinical monitoring. The display is placed toward the foot of the operating room table and is directly visible to the interventional pulmonologist and the anesthesiologist

different ventilation techniques should be available. The OR should have enough infusion pumps to administer total intravenous anesthesia (TIVA) and other supplemental infusions (e.g., carrier fluid and vasopressor). Infusion pumps are important to reduce the task load of the anesthetist in the room. The use of processed EEG monitoring (e.g., Sed Line, BIS, Entropy) to monitor the depth of anesthesia and guide anesthetic administration is strongly recommended [2, 20, 21], particularly in the absence of target-controlled infusion pumps. A bite block or tooth guard protects the teeth from dental injury and aspiration during rigid bronchoscopy [2]. Monitoring end-tidal carbon dioxide (ETCO2) is mandatory, but jet ventilation may preclude it. In cases where ETCO2 is necessary (e.g., pulmonary hypertension), conventional modes may be considered. Shared display of monitoring and bronchoscopy benefits the pulmonologist and the anesthesiologist equally (Fig. 4.3).

4.4 Modes of Ventilation

Ventilation strategies that can be used during rigid bronchoscopy include spontaneous ventilation, apneic oxygenation, conventional mechanical ventilation (spontaneous-assisted or controlled), manual jet ventilation, and mechanical jet ventilation (high or low frequency) [19, 22]. The most important premise is that patients with airway obstruction need long expiratory times. In addition, high respiratory rates risk lung overinflation, inadequate oxygenation/ventilation, and hemodynamic compromise. Thus, we recommend a normal to low respiratory rate, which may require larger tidal volumes to maintain minute ventilation. Ensuring adequate spontaneous ventilation under anesthesia through the bronchoscope may not always be feasible [2]. In our experience, controlled ventilation (jet or conventional) is routinely preferred as it allows still conditions, reducing the risk of complications. Among controlled ventilation modes, the decision is typically between volume or pressure-controlled ventilation and jet ventilation. Although challenging, spontaneous ventilation may still be applied for short procedures or under conscious sedation with vigilant monitoring [2].

Conventional ventilation can be achieved by connecting the ventilator circuit to the side port of the rigid bronchoscope with the rigid bronchoscope acting like an endotracheal tube to deliver positive pressure ventilation. Monitoring for chest rise and $ETCO_2$ is essential as displayed tidal volumes may not be accurate [23]. Different rigid bronchoscope ports are capped to reduce the amount of air leakage and the throat is usually packed with saline-soaked gauze (Fig. 4.4) [9]. When used, the number of gauzes used should be accounted for at the end of the procedure [2]. Since achieving a perfect seal is not always guaranteed, higher positive pressure breaths should be expected. Unexpected leaks, the removal and insertion of airway instruments, and deliberate apneic episodes may call for manual bag-valve ventilation. The overall limitations of manual ventilation are operator fatigue and the possibility of variable FiO_2 due to the need to rely on the reservoir bag, whose FiO_2 is affected by the previous flows and FiO_2 [23]. When using this mode of ventilation, particular attention should be paid to patients with subglottic or proximal tracheal stenosis since crossing the narrowed segment of the airway with the rigid bronchoscope is not always feasible, and successful delivery of adequate tidal volumes through the stenotic airway becomes very critical [9].

Jet ventilation uses a high-pressure gas source and applies it to an open airway in small bursts via a small catheter [23]. As explained by Ihra and Aloy, the jet injector and the stream record positive pressures during jet application. In contrast, the trachea surrounding the jet injector records sub-atmospheric pressures during each jet pulse, but not in between them. The net effect is a second stream of gas generated by air entrainment from the atmosphere, where the applied tidal volume is larger than that generated by the jet volumes alone [24]. Air entrainment alone does not explain lung expansion; the high-velocity jet stream with its forward bulk airflow is the principal mechanism. Jet ventilation during rigid bronchoscopy necessitates an open system for air entrainment, but also to relieve excess pressures. Otherwise, jet pressures will equilibrate in the alveoli and may cause barotrauma [25].

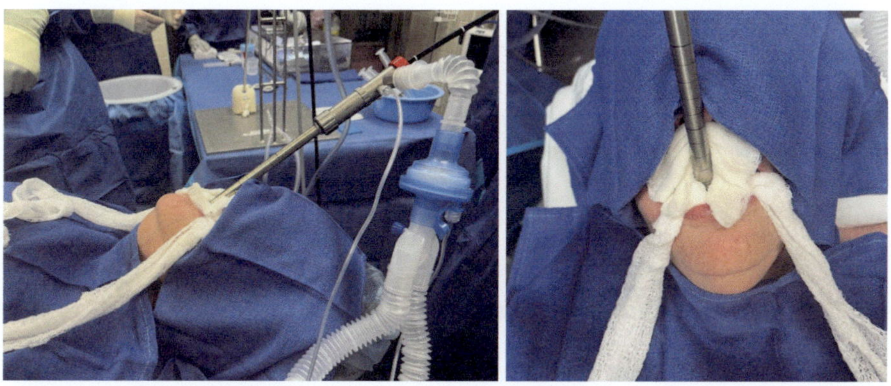

Fig. 4.4 Oropharyngeal packing during rigid bronchoscopy. Dual end-tidal monitoring from the bronchoscope and the breathing circuit, itself connected to the side port of the bronchoscope to deliver conventional mechanical ventilation

For manual jet ventilation, the gas source is high-pressure oxygen delivered at a pressure-limiting device of 50 pounds per square inch (psi) with a respiratory rate (RR) between 10 and 14. Monitoring tidal volumes becomes difficult because it is an open system and the unpredictable entrapment of ambient air [23]. Monitoring chest rise and oxygen saturations determines the adequacy of oxygenation and ventilation [22]. In an automated mechanical jet ventilator, both low- and high-frequency jet ventilation can be achieved. In a high-frequency mode, high respiratory rates (60–300 breaths/min) and low tidal volumes are delivered while the operator controls the driving pressure, inspiratory time, frequency, FiO_2, and humidification of inspired oxygen to maintain adequate oxygenation [23]. It is also equipped with an alarm system to protect against barotrauma [2]. This allows for a nearly motionless field where arterial tension of carbon dioxide can be monitored by repeated arterial blood gas measurements or by transcutaneous capnography monitoring [26, 27].

Until today, there remains no clear evidence to support either mode of ventilation. Therefore, the choice of ventilation mode relies on the preference and experience of both the anesthesiologist and bronchoscopist [8]. Nonetheless, patient's comorbidities also play a factor. For example, conventional ventilation may be preferred for patients with pulmonary hypertension since the high mean airway pressures that accompany jet ventilation could result in undesirable hemodynamic effects [2]. On the other hand, patients with interstitial lung disease have decreased lung compliance. Therefore, jet ventilation may improve oxygenation by recruiting unventilated lung zones. Barotrauma is an uncommon but well-described complication of jet ventilation that can manifest as pneumothorax, pneumomediastinum, or subcutaneous emphysema [28, 29]. Most of these complications have been described during transtracheal rather than transglottic jet ventilation [30].

4.5 Anesthetic Management

The choice of anesthetics depends on the exact procedure and the ventilation strategy to maintain oxygenation and ventilation at all times [3]. The anesthesiologist and bronchoscopist will share the airway. Therefore, mutual understanding and cooperation are crucial [3]. Sustaining hemodynamic stability, decreasing the risk of cough, laryngospasm, and airway fire while ensuring that the patient tolerates the stimulating procedure and recovers adequately from it make the anesthetic aspects of this environment even more delicate [2].

4.5.1 Moderate Sedation Versus General Anesthesia

While many simple procedures are doable under moderate sedation, general anesthesia can provide superior conditions for the proceduralist, making necessary interventions easier and faster to perform [9]. Rigid bronchoscopy is by far more stimulating than flexible bronchoscopy. Therefore, general anesthesia is almost always required [1]. Usually, the use of inhalational anesthetic is avoided to prevent contamination of the endoscopy suite with volatile agents, even with gauzes used to pack the throat [3]. In addition, the air leak impedes the accurate assessment of inhaled anesthetic delivery and true end-tidal inhaled anesthetic concentrations.

To achieve the main goals of appropriate anesthetic depth and fast recovery, the most used anesthetic technique has been total intravenous anesthesia (TIVA). That constitutes continuous infusions of propofol (50–200mcg/kg/min) with or without remifentanil (0.05–0.5 mcg/kg/min) [31]. Additional boluses may be used to suppress hemodynamic responses and laryngospasm while manipulating the rigid bronchoscope [1]. Remifentanil is useful because of its synergistic effect with propofol in achieving hypnosis and immobility [32]. As an opioid, suppression of the cough reflex is also useful during airway procedures. Its short context-sensitive half-life reduces the risk of prolonged sedation after long procedures. Moreover, it has been shown that using a higher dose of remifentanil 0.2 mcg/kg/min compared to 0.1 mcg/kg/min was well tolerated and shortened recovery time in both adults and children undergoing rigid bronchoscopy [33, 34]. Titration of infusions may be aided by using processed EEG technology [35].

Other anesthetic alternatives have been described, such as short-acting benzodiazepines like midazolam, opioids such as fentanyl and alfentanil, as well as a dexmedetomidine infusion. Remimazolam is a new ultra-short-acting benzodiazepine with faster recovery profiles than midazolam and is likely on par with propofol. While only approved for short procedures in the United States, a recent trial compared remimazolam-flumazenil with propofol in rigid bronchoscopy [36, 37]. For foreign body removal in children, dexmedetomidine was demonstrated to prolong stay in PACU although it provided appropriate anesthetic depth and hemodynamic stability in children [38]. In the elderly, dexmedetomidine can lead to a more pronounced hemodynamic depression [39].

The use of ketamine has been described in patients with hemodynamic instability as well as in patients required to maintain spontaneous ventilation. The respiratory depression and hypotension that can result from using propofol were counteracted by ketamine for therapeutic rigid bronchoscopy in patients with central airway obstruction (CAO) [40, 41]. However, adding ketamine to remifentanil-based TIVA did not provide a hemodynamic advantage compared to remifentanil and propofol [42]. The administration of muscle relaxants has multiple indications during rigid bronchoscopy. On induction, it facilitates the insertion of the rigid bronchoscope. During the maintenance phase, it provides a margin of safety from the cough reflex during delicate airway manipulation [3]. Both depolarizing and nondepolarizing NMBA have been described. The use of low-dose rocuronium for intubation has been found to provide better patient satisfaction and less postoperative myalgias than succinylcholine at the cost of inferior intubating conditions [43]. In some cases, the use of neuromuscular blocking agents has been avoided when spontaneous ventilation is preferred including airway obstruction by foreign body or central mass [3].

In addition to intravenous sedation, airway topicalization has been described. It can minimize airway response to tracheal manipulation in both children and adults [3, 44]. Lastly, complete reversal of muscle relaxation is fundamental to avoid postprocedure pulmonary complications in the setting of low pulmonary reserve in this patient population [45, 46]. Commonly, a laryngeal mask airway (LMA) and bag-valve-mask ventilation are used transiently until emergence from anesthesia [3]. The placement of an LMA facilitates ventilatory support after rigid scope removal [31].

4.6 Postoperative Care

After the emergence of anesthesia, the destination postoperatively depends on the patient's hemodynamics and intraoperative course. For uneventful, elective procedures, patients are transported to the post anesthesia care unit (PACU). Recovery encompasses raising the head of the bed and administering high FiO_2 with humidified oxygen to reduce coughing and respiratory distress [1]. Nebulized lidocaine has been found to be beneficial in addition to bronchodilators if coughing and wheezing is noted [90]. In PACU, patients are monitored for signs of respiratory distress that can occur due to hypercarbia. Patients who underwent endobronchial valve placement for bronchoscopic lung volume reduction (BLVR) routinely undergo a postoperative chest x-ray (CXR) to exclude a procedure-related pneumothorax. For procedures such as airway stent placement, a baseline CXR is needed to allow future radiographic evaluation for stent migration. Patients with high-risk airway obstruction who underwent recanalization tend to be more commonly monitored in the intensive care unit. Possible complications related to stent placement are stent migration or fracture and even central airway obstruction necessitating urgent rigid bronchoscopy to relieve the obstruction [90]. Tracheal reintubation and conventional ventilation are recommended.

4.7 Special Considerations

4.7.1 Central Airway Obstruction

Central airway obstruction (CAO) constitutes one of the most frequent indications for rigid bronchoscopy [47]. Common malignant etiologies include primary bronchogenic carcinoma, metastatic carcinoma to the airway, and mediastinal tumors [48]. Nonmalignant etiologies include post-intubation and post-tracheostomy tracheal stenosis, followed by the presence of foreign bodies, benign endobronchial tumors, and tracheobronchomalacia [49]. Stenosis of post-lung transplant anastomosis has been an emerging etiology [8]. The nature and severity of the symptoms associated with CAO depend on the anatomical structures being affected [50]. Table 4.2 explains symptoms and management considerations according to the compressed anatomical structure.

Airway collapse is a potential acute complication of anesthesia induction. The combination of supine position, induction of general anesthesia, and

Table 4.2 Symptoms, intraoperative manifestations, and special considerations according to the anatomical structure affected by compression

Anatomical structure affected	Symptoms	Possible intraoperative manifestations	Special considerations
Tracheobronchial	Stridor Dyspnea Orthopnea Chronic cough Recurrent bronchopneumonia Atelectasis Vocal cord paralysis (if RLN compressed)	Complete/partial airway collapse	Awake fiberoptic intubation
		Hypoxia Elevated peak pressures	Spontaneous ventilation
		Difficulty to ventilate/ oxygenate	Discussion of ventilation strategies distal to obstruction
Superior vena cava (SVC)	Dyspnea Headache, central nervous system symptoms Dilated collateral veins and edema in head, neck, and arms	Laryngeal swelling	Induction in fowler position
		Difficulty to ventilate/intubate	Medication administration through IVC circulation
			Careful fluid administration
Right heart and pulmonary vasculature	Dyspnea Syncope on Valsalva Arrythmias	Hypotension Hypoxemia Ca rdiocirculatory arrest	Discuss the need for extracorporeal life support due to myocardial function depression and risk of death on induction

RLN recurrent laryngeal nerve, *IVC* inferior vena cava [98, 99]

positive pressure ventilation leads to the loss of normal transpulmonary pressure gradient [50]. Moreover, relaxation of the chest wall and the bronchial smooth muscle, and the reduction in thoracic volume even without administration of neuromuscular blockade can worsen extrinsic compression and subsequently lead to complete airway obstruction. Therefore, maintenance of spontaneous ventilation is of utmost importance during all stages of anesthesia, especially induction, positioning, and emergence [51–54]. Rescue positioning in case of collapse should be discussed. Rapid placement of a rigid bronchoscope for ventilation and advancing past the obstruction may be used in the event of a complete collapse [50].

For patients presenting with bulky anterior mediastinal masses, significant cardiopulmonary compromise can occur during supine positioning and may worsen during induction and muscle relaxation [8, 51, 52, 55]. Therefore, all efforts to induce anesthesia in the sitting (or reverse Trendelenburg) position should be made if symptoms are worse in the supine position [50]. Patients with superior vena cava (SVC) syndrome are at risk of worsened right ventricular filling or ejection especially when they present with jugular venous distention, plethora to the head and neck as well as a drop in BP from upright to supine. If SVC syndrome is a concern, a pre-induction arterial line and a lower extremity intravenous access should be strongly considered [50].

4.7.2 Tumor Debulking and Thermal Ablation

Tumor debulking through the rigid bronchoscope is conducted during the management of malignant CAO with endoluminal involvement (intrinsic) [56] and mixed obstruction [8]. Endobronchial debulking can be achieved mechanically or with the use of thermal ablative techniques such as laser therapy and electrocautery therapy, including argon plasma coagulation [8]. Mechanical debulking techniques include rigid "coring" of the tumor with the tip of the rigid bronchoscope, microdebridement, or through flexible and rigid forceps. Anesthesia considerations include attention to oxygenation and ventilation in the event of significant bleeding. Lowering the FiO_2 and holding ventilation are important measures taken to decrease the risk of airway fire during cautery and laser use.

4.7.3 Bronchoplasty

Balloon bronchoplasty is typically performed for extraluminal tumors with airway compression (extrinsic) to further assist in the relief of stenosis [8]. It proves to be effective in the management of nonmalignant tracheal stenosis [4] where the radial force from the balloon is directed towards the stiffer walls of the trachea [4]. Maintaining patient immobility during balloon insufflation is essential to efficiently perform the therapeutic maneuver. When balloon bronchoplasty is conducted in the trachea, it is important to hold ventilation until the balloon has been deflated.

4.7.4 Airway Stenting

The main indication for airway stent insertion is to maintain airway patency when the residual luminal narrowing following the endobronchial intervention (tissue debulking and balloon bronchoplasty) remains flow-limiting or when the risk of recurrence of airway obstruction is significant. Stents can also cover airway defects such as in anastomotic dehiscence and tracheo-broncho-esophageal fistulas (TEF), or for excessive dynamic airway collapse and tracheo-bronchomalacia [4]. Rigid bronchoscopes are particularly useful in the placement of T-tubes, and metal and silicone stents.

General anesthesia is often performed to provide better operating conditions for the bronchoscopist as well as a more comfortable experience for the patient [50]. Patient immobility is crucial during stent deployment to avoid undesired stent displacement [50]. Constant adjustment to optimize the patient's oxygenation and ventilation is paramount. It may be prudent to avoid positive pressure ventilation in situations like TEF due to gastric insufflation and loss of tidal volume into the stomach [50].

Special attention is necessary for patients presenting with tracheal stenosis. Laryngotracheal stenosis is characterized by the narrowing of the upper airway and can occur at any level within the larynx and trachea. This narrowing can be caused by various etiologies with post-traumatic, postintubation, and post-intubation tracheal stenosis being the most common [57]. Tracheal stenting for symptomatic stenosis is usually reserved for inoperable lesions [58]. Tracheal stenting via a rigid bronchoscopy is also indicated in patients with critical airway stenosis who present with stridor [59]. The optimal method for inducing anesthesia in these patients is controversial [56]. Intravenous induction and rapid-acting muscle relaxation are likely appropriate in fixed obstructions. Manual positive pressure ventilation (PPV) improves airflow across the restriction [56]. Nouraei et al. found that muscle relaxation and positive-pressure ventilation through an LMA were effective in patients with laryngotracheal stenosis. Spontaneous ventilation creates negative inspiratory intratracheal pressure that exacerbates the gradient across an extrathoracic lesion. In contrast, positive-pressure ventilation generates positive intratracheal pressure that improves ventilation [56]. Other ventilation strategies for intraoperative ventilation include jet ventilation and HFJV [60].

4.7.5 Massive Hemoptysis

Airway hemorrhage can be a life-threatening presentation of proximal or distal airway bleeding [50]. Bleeding can occur from lung cancer, bronchiectasis, infections, or during therapeutic bronchoscopies [8]. Transbronchial lung biopsy is an independent risk factor for bleeding. When massive bleeding occurs, airway hemorrhage is more likely to cause death by asphyxiation than blood loss [50]. Therefore, lung isolation and control of bleeding become the two most critical steps. A rigid bronchoscope can help directly tamponade the site of bleeding [4]. It also allows for volume suction, preservation of adequate ventilation, and isolation of bleeding by selectively intubating the main stem bronchus [61, 62]. Due to these advantages, many bronchoscopists prefer rigid over flexible bronchoscopy for transbronchial cryo-biopsies that can bleed significantly [4]. As for lung isolation, it is crucial to protect the nonbleeding lung to prevent further worsening of gas exchange from blood spilling. Therefore, positioning the patient with the nonbleeding side up can decrease the risk of contamination [50]. A large single-lumen ETT (8.0 mm or greater) allows passage of a large therapeutic bronchoscope with high suction capability as opposed to the double-lumen tube with smaller inner diameters [63, 64]. Once the patient is stabilized, bronchial artery embolization can be considered [65, 66]. As a last resort, ECMO can be utilized in cases of severe refractory and life-threatening hypoxemia [67]. The ECMO team and thoracic surgeon should be immediately notified.

4.7.6 Foreign Body (FB) Removal

Foreign body (FB) aspiration is more common in children than in adults. Data from the National Security Council reported that about 80% of cases occur in patients younger than 15 years. Presenting symptoms vary depending on the exact location, duration of time, and type of object aspirated [68]. In adults, cough is the most common [4]. Physical exam may include wheezing [69], decreased breath sounds, retractions, and fever [4]. Radiographic imaging may help establish diagnosis but can also be normal as the majority of FBs are radiolucent [70]. The detection accuracy of FBs by plain radiography ranges from 40% to 70% [70]. Radiographic signs may include atelectasis, pulmonary infiltrates, unilateral hyperinflation, and a radiopaque FB [70]. Emphysema and infiltration are more common in distal airway obstruction [68]. Although flexible bronchoscopy can be successful in removing FBs [71, 72], rigid bronchoscopy is the gold standard [73], especially in children. Nevertheless, rigid bronchoscopy has been used in conjunction with flexible bronchoscopy [4, 70].

Anesthetic strategies focus primarily on maintaining oxygenation and avoiding displacement of the foreign body [68]. Positive pressure ventilation on induction can convert a partial obstruction into a total one by pushing the foreign body distally. Therefore, a common approach with proximal foreign body aspirations is to use inhalational induction or a cautious intravenous induction while maintaining spontaneous ventilation [68, 74]. Specific methods of general anesthesia in literature differ but the main principles are the same: maintaining hemodynamic stability, blunting airway reflexes, as well as preventing movement. If using an inhalational anesthetic, sevoflurane is generally preferred for faster induction and less airway irritation [75].

In both children and adults, TIVA with short-acting agents has been recommended [76]. A continuous propofol infusion has been successfully done with remifentanil infusion or dexmedetomidine [3, 77]. Typically, hemodynamic parameters guide titration for these infusions. In a Cochrane review, a remifentanil 0.2 μg/kg/min infusion with propofol provided hemodynamic stability and early recovery in children undergoing foreign body removal during rigid bronchoscopy [33]. However, lower doses may be required for elderly patients or patients with hemodynamic compromise [39]. A different approach used a heated high-flow nasal cannula and induction with fentanyl, intermittent propofol injection, and succinylcholine in 11 patients undergoing FB removal by rigid bronchoscopy. This approach was reported to prevent excessive coughing, irritation, and movement of the patient, vocal cords, and posterior tracheal wall as well as increase apnea time to 6 min [78].

4.7.7 Bronchoscopic Lung Volume Reduction (BLVR)

BLVR is considered for patients with advanced emphysema and hyperinflation to improve dyspnea and exercise tolerance, often refractory to medical management [79–82]. It consists of deploying one-way endobronchial valves that allow air to escape the target lobe but not re-enter, causing atelectasis of the emphysematous lung distal to the valve [79]. Generally, these patients are preoxygenated in a semi-recumbent position if dyspneic and moved to a supine position for intubation. General anesthesia with TIVA has been a preferred technique of choice, although monitored anesthesia care (MAC) with airway topicalization can also be used [83]. Other anesthesia considerations include setting longer exhalation times to avoid air trapping and avoid increases in pulmonary vascular resistance [50]. Using a more profound depth of anesthesia, 4–6 ml/kg tidal volumes, and lower positive end-expiratory pressures can help avoid the worsening of right ventricular function in these patients [50].

Pneumothorax is a major postoperative concern for BLVR procedures that can be detected postoperatively by a CXR [83]. In the absence of tension, a small pneumothorax can be carefully monitored while chest drains are reserved for larger ones [83].

4.7.8 Whole Lung Lavage

Bronchopulmonary lavage is a technique that was first described in 1966 by Ramirez-Rivera as a treatment modality for pulmonary alveolar proteinosis (PAP) [84]. It consists of irrigating one lung at a time with a large volume of saline fluid while the other lung is isolated and ventilated with 100% FiO_2. PAP is an uncommon lung disease characterized by excessive intra-alveolar accumulation of pulmonary surfactant due to autoantibodies against pulmonary granulocyte-macrophage colony-stimulating factor (GM-CSF) [85]. Patients presenting to the OR for this procedure are acutely ill with profound hypoxemia requiring invasive mechanical ventilation and even veno-venous extracorporeal membrane oxygenation (VV-ECMO). After induction of anesthesia, a left-sided double-lumen endotracheal tube is preferred for lung isolation. Positioning can be supine or decubitus. Standard ASA monitors are supplemented with an arterial line for ABG monitoring. Maintaining normothermia is important as patients are prone to becoming hypothermic after lavage with more than 10 liters of saline [86]. Airway pressure, lung compliance, and tidal volumes should be closely monitored with constant communication with the bronchoscopist [86]. Frequent airway inspection with the bronchoscope helps assess for any water leak into the ventilated lung, which is then addressed by immediate suctioning and removal of the excess fluid [85]. Hypoxemia is the main adverse effect during lung lavage procedures. Increasing FiO_2 and improving V/Q mismatch can improve oxygenation levels [85]. Positioning the ventilated lung in the dependent position during the drainage phase has been shown to decrease shunt fraction and mitigate hypoxia [87]. Avoiding high PEEP during this phase will improve compliance and decrease pulmonary vascular resistance, thus decreasing blood flow to the nonventilated lung. Concomitant use of VV ECMO, nitric oxide, and pulmonary artery occlusion of the nonventilated lung have all been described during lung lavage [88–90]. Postoperatively, controlled ventilation for alveolar recruitment is usually done in the intensive care unit.

4.7.9 Extracorporeal Membrane Oxygenation

For over four decades, extracorporeal membrane oxygenation (ECMO) has been utilized to manage cardiac and respiratory failure. Extracorporeal life support (ECLS) has a role in different types of respiratory failure, including acute respiratory distress syndrome (ARDS), decompensated pulmonary hypertension, bridge to lung transplantation, and primary graft dysfunction after lung transplantation [91]. Veno-venous (VV)-ECMO is implemented for patients with severe respiratory failure but whose cardiac function has not yet failed due to hypoxia. It is a process that takes time to set up and establish cannulation and may not be available in all hospitals. Nevertheless, it has also been successfully used in critical airway situations where airway loss was imminent [92, 93]. VV-ECMO can provide a respiratory support tool perioperatively and accompany other methods of restoring the airway. An example of that is patients who are at risk of life-threatening external airway compression from anterior mediastinal masses [94]. These patients can be at risk of profound hypoxemia and hypercapnia due to airway obstruction. Other examples include tracheal reconstruction and whole lung lavage as mentioned in previous sections [93]. A venoarterial ECMO can also support circulation in extreme cases.

4.8 Complications

Preoperative assessment, preparation, planning, and expertise can significantly reduce complications after rigid bronchoscopy [4]. Overall, the complication rate averages 3.9% [95]. However, rates have been reported between 0.9% and 11.7%. The ACCS AQuire registry published the results of a large, prospective study on therapeutic bronchoscopy for central airway obstruction. Emergent procedures, ASA>3, re-do bronchoscopy, and moderate sedation were found to be risk factors for complications [95].

The most common postoperative complaints include sore throat and sore neck. Injury to the oropharynx, airway, and glottic structures is also possible [2]. Dental injury can be avoided by careful dental examination preprocedure. More serious complications are encountered in patients with significant comorbidities. These include bronchospasm, laryngospasm, bleeding, airway perforation, airway fires, and pneumothorax [2]. Periprocedural mortality rates are generally lower than 0.5% [95]. Hypoxemia-induced cardiac ischemia and arrhythmia may occur due to the hypoxic and apneic periods during the procedure [4, 96, 97]. Intraoperative hypoxemia was associated with tracheal stenosis of more than 75%, tumor removal procedures, ASA 4, and baseline oxygen saturation of less than 96% [96]. Refractory hypoxemia, although uncommon (2%), was associated with redo bronchoscopy, tracheoesophageal fistula repair, and moderate sedation [95]. Similarly, unexpected respiratory failure within 24 h had an incidence of 1.3% and was associated with ASA>3, hematologic malignancy, left mainstem disease, and electrocautery.

4.9 Conclusion

Anesthesia for rigid bronchoscopy and bronchial interventions requires a deep understanding of the pathophysiology of the disease process being treated and preoperative and intraoperative recognition of the altered physiologic and hemodynamic parameters. A tailored and patient-specific anesthesia management plan is recommended with special consideration to the nature of the disease process being treated and the preexisting cardiopulmonary reserve. Proper and constant communication between the anesthesia and the interventional pulmonology teams is key to any therapeutic rigid bronchoscopy procedure. Readiness, alertness, and anticipatory behavior constitute essential team attributes to ensure success.

References

1. de Lima A, Kheir F, Majid A, Pawlowski J. Anesthesia for interventional pulmonology procedures: a review of advanced diagnostic and therapeutic bronchoscopy. Can J Anaesth. 2018;65(7):822–36.
2. Goudra BG, Singh PM, Borle A, Farid N, Harris K. Anesthesia for advanced Bronchoscopic procedures: state-of-the-art review. Lung. 2015;193(4):453–65.
3. José RJ, Shaefi S, Navani N. Anesthesia for bronchoscopy. Curr Opin Anesthesiol. 2014;27(4):453–7.
4. Batra H, Yarmus L. Indications and complications of rigid bronchoscopy. Expert Rev Respir Med. 2018;12(6):509–20.
5. Zöllner F. Gustav Killian, father of bronchoscopy. Arch Otolaryngol. 1965;82(6):656–9.
6. Panchabhai TS, Mehta AC. Historical perspectives of bronchoscopy. Connecting the dots. Ann Am Thorac Soc. 2015;12(5):631–41.
7. Aravena C, Mehta AC, Almeida FA, Lamb C, Maldonado F, Gildea TR. Innovation in rigid bronchoscopy—past, present, and future. J Thorac Dis. 2023;15(5):2836–47.
8. Diaz-Mendoza J, Peralta AR, Debiane L, Simoff MJ. Rigid bronchoscopy. Semin Respir Crit Care Med. 2018;39(06):674–84.
9. Abdelmalak BB, Doyle DJ. Updates and controversies in anesthesia for advanced interventional pulmonology procedures. Curr Opin Anaesthesiol. 2021;34(4):455–63.
10. Sarkiss M. Anesthesia for bronchoscopy and interventional pulmonology: from moderate sedation to jet ventilation. Curr Opin Pulm Med. 2011;17(4):274–8.
11. Duffy JR, Litts JK, Fink DS. Superior laryngeal nerve block for treatment of neurogenic cough. Laryngoscope. 2021;131(10):E2676–e80.
12. Plaza-Lloret M, González-López L, Mínguez-Marín CA, López-Rincón RM. Ultrasound-guided superior laryngeal nerve block for rigid bronchoscopy. Rev Esp Anestesiol Reanim. 2015;62(3):174–6.
13. Nicastri D, Weiser T. Rigid bronchoscopy: indications and techniques. Oper Tech Thorac Cardiovasc Surg. 2012;17:44–51.
14. Malik JA, Gupta D, Agarwal AN, Jindal SK. Anticholinergic premedication for flexible bronchoscopy: a randomized, double-blind, placebo-controlled study of atropine and glycopyrrolate. Chest. 2009;136(2):347–54.
15. Wahidi MM, Jain P, Jantz M, Lee P, Mackensen GB, Barbour SY, et al. American College of Chest Physicians consensus statement on the use of topical anesthesia, analgesia, and sedation during flexible bronchoscopy in adult patients. Chest. 2011;140(5):1342–50.
16. Suhre WM, Lang JD Jr, Madtes DK, Abdelmalak BB. Partnership with interventional pulmonologist: an anesthesiologist's perspective. Otolaryngol Clin N Am. 2019;52(6):1049–63.
17. Woerlee GM. Preoperative assessment of respiratory function & its consequences. In: Common perioperative problems and the anaesthetist. Dordrecht: Springer Netherlands; 1988. p. 179–89.
18. Degani-Costa LH, Faresin SM, dos Reis Falcão LF. Preoperative evaluation of the patient with pulmonary disease. Braz J Anesthesiol (Engl Ed). 2014;64(1):22–34.
19. Beamis JF, Becker HD, Cavaliere S, Colt H, Diaz-Jimenez JP, Dumon JF, et al. ERS/ATS statement on interventional pulmonology. Chairmen: CT Bolliger, PN Mathur. Eur Respir J. 2002;19(2):356–73.

20. Whitlock EL, Villafranca AJ, Lin N, Palanca BJ, Jacobsohn E, Finkel KJ, et al. Relationship between bispectral index values and volatile anesthetic concentrations during the maintenance phase of anesthesia in the B-Unaware trial. Anesthesiology. 2011;115(6):1209–18.
21. Yamada J, Hazama D, Tachihara M, Kawanami Y, Kawaguchi A, Yatani A, et al. The utility of bispectral index monitoring in flexible bronchoscopy: a single-center, retrospective observational study. Thorac Cancer. 2022;13(21):3052–7.
22. Pathak V, Welsby I, Mahmood K, Wahidi M, MacIntyre N, Shofer S. Ventilation and anesthetic approaches for rigid bronchoscopy. Ann Am Thorac Soc. 2014;11(4):628–34.
23. Chadha M, Kulshrestha M, Biyani A. Anaesthesia for bronchoscopy. Indian J Anaesth. 2015;59(9):565–73.
24. Ihra G, Aloy A. On the use of Venturi's principle to describe entrainment during jet ventilation. J Clin Anesth. 2000;12(5):417–9.
25. Spoerel WE, Narayanan PS, Singh NP. Transtracheal ventilation. Br J Anaesth. 1971;43(10):932–9.
26. Biro P, Layer M, Wiedemann K, Seifert B, Spahn DR. Carbon dioxide elimination during high-frequency jet ventilation for rigid bronchoscopy. Br J Anaesth. 2000;84(5):635–7.
27. Principi T, Pantanetti S, Elisei D, Strovegli D, Gasparini S, Pelaia P. Carbon dioxide monitoring during high-frequency jet ventilation for rigid bronchoscopy. Crit Care. 2003;7(2):P159.
28. Benumof Jonathan L, Gaughan Sheila D. Concerns regarding barotrauma during jet ventilation. Anesthesiology. 1992;76(6):1072.
29. Clevenger FW, Acosta JA, Osler TM, Demarest GB, Fry DE. Barotrauma associated with high-frequency jet ventilation for hypoxic salvage. Arch Surg. 1990;125(12):1542–5.
30. Jaquet Y, Monnier P, Van Melle G, Ravussin P, Spahn Donat R, Chollet-Rivier M. Complications of different ventilation strategies in endoscopic laryngeal surgery: a 10-year review. Anesthesiology. 2006;104(1):52–9.
31. José RJ, Shaefi S, Navani N. Anesthesia for bronchoscopy. Curr Opin Anaesthesiol. 2014;27(4):453–7.
32. Hendrickx JF, Eger EI 2nd, Sonner JM, Shafer SL. Is synergy the rule? A review of anesthetic interactions producing hypnosis and immobility. Anesth Analg. 2008;107(2):494–506.
33. Teksan L, Baris S, Karakaya D, Dilek A. A dose study of remifentanil in combination with propofol during tracheobronchial foreign body removal in children. J Clin Anesth. 2013;25(3):198–201.
34. Goudra BG, Singh PM, Manjunath AK, Reihmer JW, Haas AR, Lanfranco AR, et al. Effectiveness of high dose remifentanil in preventing coughing and laryngospasm in non-paralyzed patients for advanced bronchoscopic procedures. Ann Thorac Med. 2014;9(1):23–8.
35. Myles PS, Leslie K, McNeil J, Forbes A, Chan MT. Bispectral index monitoring to prevent awareness during anaesthesia: the B-aware randomised controlled trial. Lancet. 2004;363(9423):1757–63.
36. Pan Y, Chen M, Gu F, Chen J, Zhang W, Huang Z, et al. Comparison of remimazolam-flumazenil versus propofol for rigid bronchoscopy: a prospective randomized controlled trial. J Clin Med. 2022;12(1):257.
37. Wu Q, Xu R, Zhou X, Wang L, Sheng C, Ding M, et al. Bolus administration of remimazolam was superior to midazolam for deep sedation in elderly patients undergoing diagnostic bronchoscopy: a randomized, double-blind, controlled trial. Medicine (Baltimore). 2024;103(12):e37215.
38. Cai Y, Li W, Chen K. Efficacy and safety of spontaneous ventilation technique using dexmedetomidine for rigid bronchoscopic airway foreign body removal in children. Paediatr Anaesth. 2013;23(11):1048–53.
39. Chen K, Shen X. Dexmedetomidine and propofol total intravenous anesthesia for airway foreign body removal. Irish Journal of Medical Science (1971 -). 2014;183(3):481–4.
40. Gupta N, Dutta K, Garg R, Bharti SJ. Ketamine and propofol infusion for therapeutic rigid bronchoscopy in a patient with central airway obstruction. J Anaesthesiol Clin Pharmacol. 2019;35(3):410–2.

41. Thakore S, Gupta N, Madan K, Bhatnagar S. Near ideal anesthetic technique for tracheal stenting in central airway obstruction with dexmedetomidine-ketamine infusion: a case report. Braz J Anesthesiol (Engl Ed). 2021;71(4):447–50.
42. Bakan M, Topuz U, Umutoglu T, Gundogdu G, Ilce Z, Elicevik M, et al. Remifentanil-based total intravenous anesthesia for pediatric rigid bronchoscopy: comparison of adjuvant propofol and ketamine. Clinics (Sao Paulo). 2014;69(6):372–7.
43. Ghezel-Ahmadi V, Ghezel-Ahmadi D, Mangen J, Bolukbas S, Welker A, Kuerschner VC, et al. Comparing patient satisfaction and intubating conditions using succinylcholine or low-dose Rocuronium for rigid bronchoscopy: a randomized study. Thorac Cardiovasc Surg. 2015;63(6):526–32.
44. Mihara T, Uchimoto K, Morita S, Goto T. The efficacy of lidocaine to prevent laryngospasm in children: a systematic review and meta-analysis. Anaesthesia. 2014;69(12):1388–96.
45. Murphy GS, Brull SJ. Residual neuromuscular block: lessons unlearned. Part I: definitions, incidence, and adverse physiologic effects of residual neuromuscular block. Anesth Analg. 2010;111(1):120–8.
46. Brull SJ, Murphy GS. Residual neuromuscular block: lessons unlearned. Part II: methods to reduce the risk of residual weakness. Anesth Analg. 2010;111(1):129–40.
47. Petrella F, Borri A, Casiraghi M, Cavaliere S, Donghi S, Galetta D, et al. Operative rigid bronchoscopy: indications, basic techniques and results. Multimed Man Cardiothorac Surg. 2014;2014:mmu006.
48. Ernst A, Feller-Kopman D, Becker HD, Mehta AC. Central airway obstruction. Am J Respir Crit Care Med. 2004;169(12):1278–97.
49. Barros Casas D, Fernández-Bussy S, Folch E, Flandes Aldeyturriaga J, Majid A. Non-malignant central airway obstruction. Arch Bronconeumol. 2014;50(8):345–54.
50. Galway U, Zura A, Khanna S, Wang M, Turan A, Ruetzler K. Anesthetic considerations for bronchoscopic procedures: a narrative review based on the Cleveland Clinic experience. J Thorac Dis. 2019;11(7):3156–70.
51. Goh MH, Liu XY, Goh YS. Anterior mediastinal masses: an anaesthetic challenge. Anaesthesia. 1999;54(7):670–4.
52. Neuman GG, Weingarten AE, Abramowitz RM, Kushins LG, Abramson AL, Ladner W. The anesthetic management of the patient with an anterior mediastinal mass. Anesthesiology. 1984;60(2):144–7.
53. Chen SH, Hsu JC, Lui PW, Chen CH, Yang CY. Airway obstruction by a metastatic mediastinal tumor during anesthesia. Chang Gung Med J. 2005;28(4):258–63.
54. Blank RS, de Souza DG. Anesthetic management of patients with an anterior mediastinal mass: continuing professional development. Can J Anaesth. 2011;58(9):853–9, 60-7.
55. Prakash UB, Abel MD, Hubmayr RD. Mediastinal mass and tracheal obstruction during general anesthesia. Mayo Clin Proc. 1988;63(10):1004–11.
56. Nouraei SAR, Giussani DA, Howard DJ, Sandhu GS, Ferguson C, Patel A. Physiological comparison of spontaneous and positive-pressure ventilation in laryngotracheal stenosis. Br J Anaesth. 2008;101(3):419–23.
57. Tsakiridis K, Darwiche K, Visouli AN, Zarogoulidis P, Machairiotis N, Christofis C, et al. Management of complex benign post-tracheostomy tracheal stenosis with bronchoscopic insertion of silicon tracheal stents, in patients with failed or contraindicated surgical reconstruction of trachea. J Thorac Dis. 2012;4(Suppl 1):32–40.
58. Puma F, Ragusa M, Avenia N, Urbani M, Droghetti A, Daddi N, et al. The role of silicone stents in the treatment of cicatricial tracheal stenoses. J Thorac Cardiovasc Surg. 2000;120(6):1064–9.
59. Espinoza A, Neumann K, Halvorsen PS, Sundset A, Kongerud J, Fosse E. Critical airway obstruction: challenges in airway management and ventilation during therapeutic bronchoscopy. J Bronchol Interv Pulmonol. 2015;22(1):41–7.
60. Wiedemann K, Männle C. Anesthesia and gas exchange in tracheal surgery. Thorac Surg Clin. 2014;24(1):13–25.
61. Casal RF. Update in airway stents. Curr Opin Pulm Med. 2010;16(4):321–8.

62. Karush JM, Seder CW, Raman A, Chmielewski GW, Liptay MJ, Warren WH, et al. Durability of silicone airway stents in the management of Benign Central Airway Obstruction. Lung. 2017;195(5):601–6.
63. Cohen E. Pro: the new bronchial blockers are preferable to double-lumen tubes for lung isolation. J Cardiothorac Vasc Anesth. 2008;22(6):920–4.
64. Klafta JM, Olson JP. Emergent lung separation for management of pulmonary artery rupture. Anesthesiology. 1997;87(5):1248–50.
65. Chen J, Chen LA, Liang ZX, Li CS, Tian Q, Yang Z, et al. Immediate and long-term results of bronchial artery embolization for hemoptysis due to benign versus malignant pulmonary diseases. Am J Med Sci. 2014;348(3):204–9.
66. Alexander GR. A retrospective review comparing the treatment outcomes of emergency lung resection for massive haemoptysis with and without preoperative bronchial artery embolization. Eur J Cardiothorac Surg. 2014;45(2):251–5.
67. Lee CF, Huang CT, Ruan SY. Endotracheal tube clamping and extracorporeal membrane oxygenation to resuscitate massive pulmonary haemorrhage. Respirol Case Rep. 2018;6(5):e00321.
68. Kendigelen P. The anaesthetic consideration of tracheobronchial foreign body aspiration in children. J Thorac Dis. 2016;8(12):3803–7.
69. Martinot A, Closset M, Marquette CH, Hue V, Deschildre A, Ramon P, et al. Indications for flexible versus rigid bronchoscopy in children with suspected foreign-body aspiration. Am J Respir Crit Care Med. 1997;155(5):1676–9.
70. Shostak E. Foreign body removal in children and adults: review of available techniques and emerging technologies. AME Med J. 2018;3:75.
71. Ramos-Rossy J, Cantres O, Torres A, Casal J, Otero Y, Arzon-Nieves G, et al. Flexible Bronchoscopic removal of 3 foreign objects. Fed Pract. 2018;35(9):24–6.
72. Kim K, Lee HJ, Yang EA, Kim HS, Chun YH, Yoon JS, et al. Foreign body removal by flexible bronchoscopy using retrieval basket in children. Ann Thorac Med. 2018;13(2):82–5.
73. Boufersaoui A, Smati L, Benhalla KN, Boukari R, Smail S, Anik K, et al. Foreign body aspiration in children: experience from 2624 patients. Int J Pediatr Otorhinolaryngol. 2013;77(10):1683–8.
74. Fidkowski CW, Zheng H, Firth PG. The anesthetic considerations of tracheobronchial foreign bodies in children: a literature review of 12,979 cases. Anesth Analg. 2010;111(4):1016–25.
75. Liao R, Li JY, Liu GY. Comparison of sevoflurane volatile induction/maintenance anaesthesia and propofol-remifentanil total intravenous anaesthesia for rigid bronchoscopy under spontaneous breathing for tracheal/bronchial foreign body removal in children. Eur J Anaesthesiol. 2010;27(11):930–4.
76. Putz L, Mayné A, Dincq A-S. Jet ventilation during rigid bronchoscopy in adults: a focused review. Biomed Res Int. 2016;2016(1):4234861.
77. Chen K, Shen X. Dexmedetomidine and propofol total intravenous anesthesia for airway foreign body removal. Ir J Med Sci. 2014;183(3):481–4.
78. Srivastava R, Pathak M, Mallan D. THIRVE in foreign body bronchus removal-a novel approach. Indian J Otolaryngol Head Neck Surg. 2021;73(3):356–9.
79. Elayaperumal AK, Jackson RE. Anaesthesia for lung volume reduction surgery and endobronchial valves. BJA Educ. 2018;18(7):193–8.
80. Strange C, Herth FJ, Kovitz KL, McLennan G, Ernst A, Goldin J, et al. Design of the Endobronchial Valve for Emphysema Palliation Trial (VENT): a non-surgical method of lung volume reduction. BMC Pulm Med. 2007;7:10.
81. Davey C, Zoumot Z, Jordan S, McNulty WH, Carr DH, Hind MD, et al. Bronchoscopic lung volume reduction with endobronchial valves for patients with heterogeneous emphysema and intact interlobar fissures (the BeLieVeR-HIFi study): a randomised controlled trial. Lancet. 2015;386(9998):1066–73.
82. Klooster K, ten Hacken NH, Hartman JE, Kerstjens HA, van Rikxoort EM, Slebos DJ. Endobronchial valves for emphysema without Interlobar collateral ventilation. N Engl J Med. 2015;373(24):2325–35.

83. Thiruvenkatarajan V, Maycock T, Grosser D, Currie J. Anaesthetic management for endobronchial valve insertion: lessons learned from a single Centre retrospective series and a literature review. BMC Anesthesiol. 2018;18(1):206.
84. Ramirez J. Bronchopulmonary lavage. New techniques and observations. Dis Chest. 1966;50(6):581–8.
85. Pandit A, Gupta N, Madan K, Bharti SJ, Kumar V. Anaesthetic considerations for whole lung lavage for pulmonary alveolar proteinosis. Ghana Med J. 2019;53(3):248–51.
86. Manohar M, Bansal P. Whole lung lavage in pulmonary alveolar proteinosis: anesthetic management and challenges. Ain-Shams J Anesthesiol. 2022;14(1):15.
87. Smith JD, Millen JE, Safar P, Robin ED. Intrathoracic pressure, pulmonary vascular pressures and gas exchange during pulmonary lavage. Anesthesiology. 1970;33(4):401–5.
88. Ben-Abraham R, Greenfeld A, Rozenman J, Ben-Dov I. Pulmonary alveolar proteinosis: step-by-step perioperative care of whole lung lavage procedure. Heart Lung. 2002;31(1):43–9.
89. Ahmed R, Iqbal M, Kashef SH, Almomatten MI. Whole lung lavage with intermittent double lung ventilation. A modified technique for managing pulmonary alveolar proteinosis. Saudi Med J. 2005;26(1):139–41.
90. Nadeau MJ, Côté D, Bussières JS. The combination of inhaled nitric oxide and pulmonary artery balloon inflation improves oxygenation during whole-lung lavage. Anesth Analg. 2004;99(3):676–9.
91. Short B, Burkart KM. Extracorporeal life support in respiratory failure. Clin Chest Med. 2022;43(3):519–28.
92. Abdelmalak BB. The role of extracorporeal membrane oxygenation in the Management of the Difficult Airway. J Cardiothorac Vasc Anesth. 2023;37(12):2660–1.
93. Wu H, Zhuo K, Cheng D. Extracorporeal membrane oxygenation in critical airway interventional therapy: a review. Front Oncol. 2023;13:1098594.
94. Pořízka M, Michálek P, Votruba J, Abdelmalak BB. Extracorporeal oxygenation techniques in adult critical airway obstruction: a review. Prague Med Rep. 2021;122(2):61–72.
95. Ost DE, Ernst A, Grosu HB, Lei X, Diaz-Mendoza J, Slade M, et al. Complications following therapeutic bronchoscopy for malignant central airway obstruction: results of the AQuIRE registry. Chest. 2015;148(2):450–71.
96. Chumpathong S, Tscheikuna J, Boonsombat T, Muangman S, Luansritisakul C. Incidence and risk factors of hypoxemia during interventional rigid bronchoscopy under spontaneous-assisted ventilation. J Bronchol Interv Pulmonol. 2017;24(4):268–74.
97. Murgu S, Laxmanan B, Stoy S, Egressy K, Chaddha U, Farooqui F, et al. Evaluation of safety and Short-term outcomes of therapeutic rigid bronchoscopy using Total intravenous anesthesia and spontaneous assisted ventilation. Respiration. 2020;99(3):239–47.
98. Rogers DJ, Cunnane MB, Hartnick CJ. Vascular compression of the airway: establishing a functional diagnostic algorithm. JAMA Otolaryngol Head Neck Surg. 2013;139(6):586–91.
99. Massullo D, Di Benedetto P, Pinto G. Intraoperative strategy in patients with extended involvement of mediastinal structures. Thorac Surg Clin. 2009;19(1):113–20.

5 Anesthesia for Endobronchial Ultrasound-Guided Transbronchial Fine Needle Aspiration

Kelly Mishra

5.1 Introduction

5.1.1 The Procedure

Endobronchial ultrasound-guided transbronchial needle aspiration (EBUS-TBNA) was introduced in 2003 and is now the standard of care for the evaluation of mediastinal and hilar lymphadenopathy [1]. In many clinical circumstances, EBUS has been able to replace mediastinoscopy and is a lower risk alternative. A linear array ultrasonic bronchoscope is utilized to perform real-time transbronchial needle aspiration with a 22 g needle under direct ultrasound guidance. A hybrid bronchoscope system is utilized that provides both ultrasound and fiberoptic imaging. The scope is inserted into the airway until the desired position is reached, then the balloon is inflated with normal saline to optimize ultrasound imaging (Fig. 5.1). Vascular landmarks and surrounding landmarks are identified with ultrasound Doppler [2]. The needle is then advanced from the scope to perform a biopsy. A lab technician is typically present in the bronchoscopy suite to examine the biopsy sample to determine if it is adequate.

5.1.2 Patient Population and Anatomic Considerations

Endobronchial ultrasound-guided transbronchial needle aspiration (EBUS-TBNA) is often utilized for lung cancer staging. It can also be used to diagnose sarcoidosis or tuberculosis. EBUS-TBNA can access the paratracheal, subcarinal, hilar, and interlobar lymph node locations. Thoracic lymph node locations that may require other modalities of biopsy are the aortopulmonary and prevascular (accessed with

K. Mishra (✉)
Vanderbilt University School of Medicine, Nashville, TN, USA
e-mail: kelly.mishra@vumc.org

M. Sarkiss (ed.), *Anesthesia for Interventional Pulmonary Procedures*,
https://doi.org/10.1007/978-3-032-12007-6_5

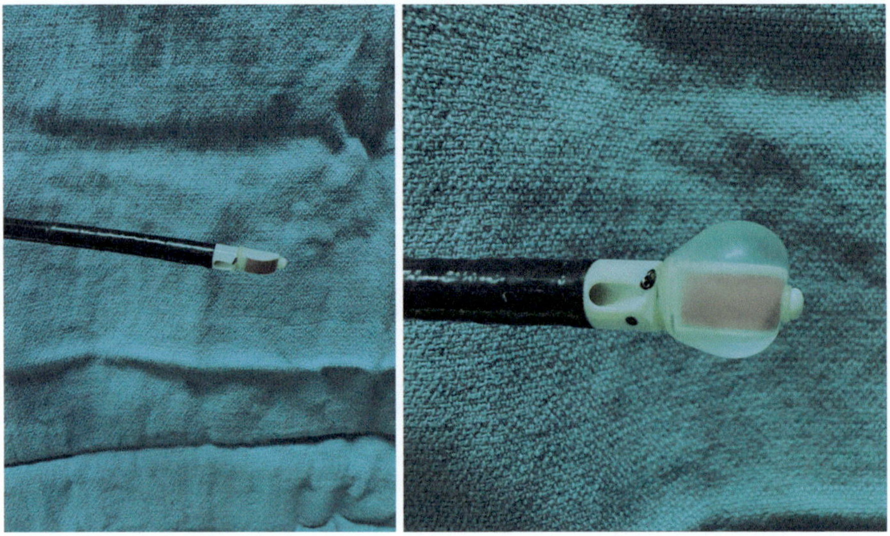

Fig. 5.1 An endobronchial ultrasound with balloon deflated and inflated

anterior mediastinoscopy) and paraesophageal (accessed with endoscopic transesopohageal ultrasound-guided fine needle aspiration), and those within the inferior pulmonary ligament [2] (Fig. 5.2).

5.1.3 Anesthetic Goals

The goals of providing anesthesia for EBUS-TBNA are patient safety, patient comfort, creating optimal procedural conditions, and minimizing complications. As with any procedure, a safely anesthetized and still patient dramatically decreases procedural and anesthetic risk. EBUS is performed with TBNA in part to be more precise and increase safety, but if a patient coughs or moves at the time the biopsy is being taken, then there is a risk of biopsy of the wrong site. Any bronchoscopy can cause a patient to cough, and this is a patient population that is likely predisposed to coughing as well, so cough suppression is an important anesthetic goal. The exception to this can be that some coughing with topicalization is expected and can help spread the lidocaine. An additional anesthetic goal is efficiency in the bronchoscopy suite. Typically, a considerable number of bronchoscopies are boarded in a room in a day. Efficient turn overs, inductions, and emergence are very important. An additional important factor that is worth noting is the importance of very close communication with the interventional pulmonologists about any airway concerns or oxygenation/ventilation issues during the case as this is a team sport and the anesthesiologist and pulmonologist are working together to manage these patients. Difficult airways are often jointly identified and managed given the combined expertise.

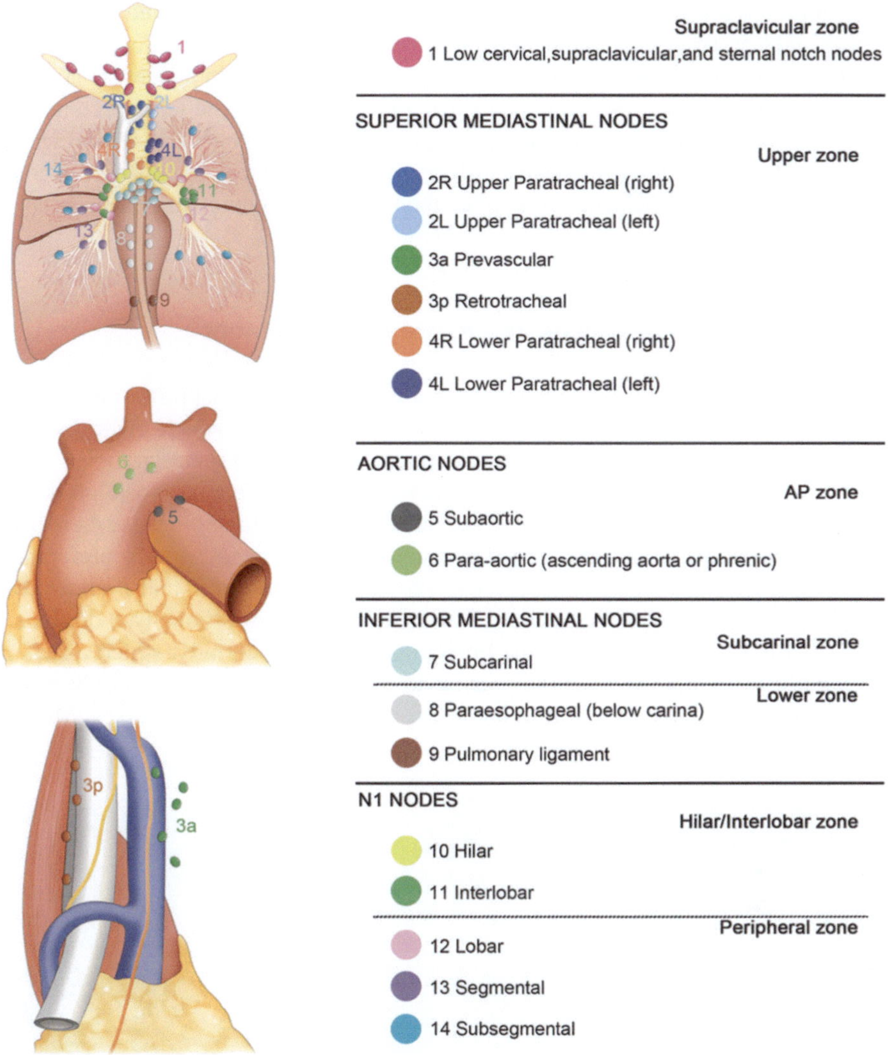

Fig. 5.2 Mountain classification of the mediastinal and hilar lymph nodes [3]

5.2 Anesthetic Considerations

5.2.1 General Goals and Choosing an Anesthetic Plan

Both general anesthesia and sedation can create safe conditions for EBUS-TBNA to be performed, and studies have not found one specific technique to be superior. The choice of anesthetic plan must consider the patient's airway exam, body habitus, and comorbidities, specifically their cardiac and respiratory status. Additionally, patient preference may play a role. Studies have not consistently found statistically significant differences in diagnostic yield, sensitivity, or major complications [4–6]. Interestingly, there have also not been significant differences in patient satisfaction [7]. Cough suppression with moderate sedation has been found to be incomplete, which might make general anesthesia preferable [5, 8]. The general logistical set-up and bronchoscopy suite also make a difference. If an anesthesiologist is involved in every case, regardless of anesthetic plan, then choosing general anesthesia is not a logistical barrier.

5.2.2 General Anesthesia and Airway Management

A major advantage of utilizing general anesthesia is that optimal procedural conditions can be created for the interventional pulmonologist, which contributes to improved diagnostic accuracy. Both endotracheal tube (ETT) and laryngeal mask airway can be acceptable choices for airway management, but laryngeal mask airway (LMA) is often the preference of the interventional pulmonologists when there are not contraindications (Fig. 5.3). There are three reasons an LMA is preferable. The large internal diameter of the LMA allows scope insertion, and it allows for access to the higher mediastinal lymph node stations [2]. Additionally, a disadvantage of an ETT is that it causes the bronchoscope to lie centrally, which makes it difficult to bring the tip close the mucosa to optimize imaging [2]. Muscle relaxation is often utilized even with a laryngeal mask airway for these cases. Muscle

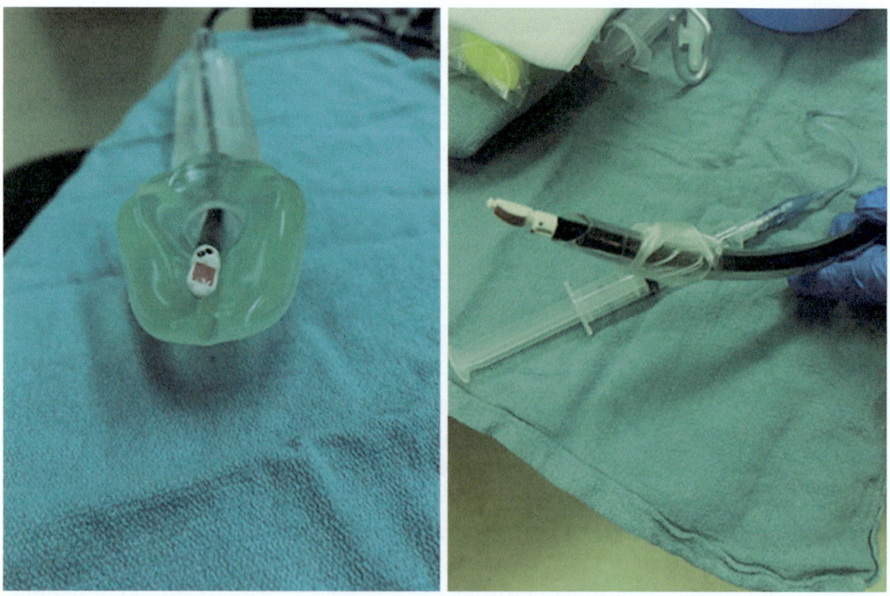

Fig. 5.3 An endobronchial ultrasound inside an LMA and an ETT

relaxation prevents reflex coughing, which can cause inadequate imaging, inaccurate insertion of the needle, and possible mediastinal vessel injury. Also, when the balloon is inflated with saline it can result in temporary airway obstruction and coughing against an occluded airway can result in negative pressure pulmonary edema [2]. If an endotracheal tube is utilized, typically an 8.5 or 9.0 ETT is required so that there is adequate space around the probe for ventilation.

Total intravenous anesthesia is utilized rather than volatile anesthesia given the unreliability of volatile delivery and the frequent suctioning of the airway [2]. Patients are typically maintained on 100% FiO2 during the procedure. The airway can become irritated with multiple scope insertions through the vocal cord or by intubation with a large ETT, and dexamethasone can minimize airway edema.

5.2.3 Conscious Sedation and Topical Anesthesia

The advantage of utilizing sedation is that it avoids utilizing an artificial airway and muscle relaxation, which has varying degrees of benefit depending on the patient's respiratory status and comorbidities. Additionally avoiding general anesthesia can have some hemodynamic benefits, which in some patient populations might be important. One study comparing moderate vs deep sedation found improved diagnostic yield in the deep sedation group, but other studies have found no difference [9, 10]. Moderate sedation can be provided in various forms such as a propofol infusion, Precedex infusion, or midazolam and fentanyl boluses. With any sedation choice for bronchoscopy, topicalization is required for both patient comfort and cough suppression. Typically, the topicalization is provided by interventional pulmonologist. As with sedation regimens, topicalization regimens can vary but an example of a topicalization algorithm would be administering nebulized 4% lidocaine during transport to the bronchoscopy suite from the holding room, having the patient gargle with 2% viscous lidocaine, administering 10 cc of 2% lidocaine above the cords with the bronchoscope (in syringes with 1 cc lidocaine and 9 cc air), and 20 cc of 1% lidocaine below the cords (again with 1 cc lidocaine and 9 cc air). For the lidocaine administration above the vocal cords, you should aim for the following structures: epiglottis, posterior arytenoids, right cord, left cord, and the anterior commissure of the vocal cords (lidocaine will drip down and hit the posterior commissure). Once the bronchoscope is through the cords, the following parts of the tracheobronchial tree should be topicalized: cricoid, anterior trachea (near aortic arch), carina, right bronchus, and left bronchus.

5.3 Complications

EBUS-TBNA is a very safe procedure with very rare complications. Complications can include pneumothorax, pneumomediastinum, and bleeding from mediastinal vessels. Thankfully the pneumothorax risk is small since the pleural space is not violated. The fact that a small gauge needle is utilized also prevents risk. The risks of anesthesia (sedation or general anesthesia) for EBUS-TBNA can vary widely depending on the patient obviously, but it is generally low risk regardless of anesthetic choice. In bronchoscopy suites without anesthesia, staffing deep sedation in the absence of anesthesiologist might increase the risk of complications [5].

5.4 Emergence and PACU Considerations

Airway stimulation during the procedure leads to excessive secretions, and this can lead to increased risks of coughing bronchospasm, and laryngospasm. Adequate suctioning prior to extubation or LMA removal is critical [2]. Patients do not typically report significant pain related to the procedure and so high doses of narcotics are not frequently needed [2]. Since this is often an outpatient procedure with only 1–2 h in the PACU, the anesthetic plan and postop orders should be in line with setting the patient up for success with an expedited PACU stay and a drive home. Since complications are rare but serious, it is especially important to be vigilant about identifying any patient who does not appear to be on pathway and working with the pulmonologist to rule out any complications such as pneumothorax.

5.5 Conclusion

Providing anesthesia for EBUS-TBNA can be "simple" if you set yourself up for success with appropriate anesthetic planning working with your interventional pulmonologists. There can be logistical, team, procedural, or patient elements that factor into the appropriate anesthetic planning. As with all procedures, and perhaps even so with airway procedures, understanding exactly what the procedure entails is critical both for planning, administering anesthesia, and responding to complications.

References

1. Vaidya PJ, Munavvar M, Leuppi JD, Mehta AC, Chhajed PN. Endobronchial ultrasound-guided transbronchial needle aspiration: safe as it sounds. Respirology. 2017;22(6):1093–101.
2. Sarkiss M, Kennedy M, Riedel B, Norman P, Morice R, Jimenez C, et al. Anesthesia technique for endobronchial ultrasound-guided fine needle aspiration of mediastinal lymph node. J Cardiothorac Vasc Anesth. 2007;21(6):892–6.
3. Ji H, Hu C, Yang X, Liu Y, Ji G, Ge S, et al. Lymph node metastasis in cancer progression: molecular mechanisms, clinical significance and therapeutic interventions. Signal Transduct Target Ther. 2023;8(1):367.
4. Wahidi MM, Jain P, Jantz M, Lee P, Mackensen GB, Barbour SY, et al. American College of Chest Physicians consensus statement on the use of topical anesthesia, analgesia, and sedation during flexible bronchoscopy in adult patients. Chest. 2011;140(5):1342–50.
5. Cornelissen CG, Dapper J, Dreher M, Muller T. Endobronchial ultrasound-guided transbronchial needle aspiration under general anesthesia versus bronchoscopist-directed deep sedation: a retrospective analysis. Endosc Ultrasound. 2019;8(3):204–8.

6. Yarmus LB, Akulian JA, Gilbert C, Mathai SC, Sathiyamoorthy S, Sahetya S, et al. Comparison of moderate versus deep sedation for endobronchial ultrasound transbronchial needle aspiration. Ann Am Thorac Soc. 2013;10(2):121–6.
7. Wahidi MM, Sterman DH. Bringing comfort to endobronchial ultrasound bronchoscopy. Am J Respir Crit Care Med. 2015;191(7):727–8.
8. Mohan A, Madan K, Hadda V, Mittal S, Suri T, Shekh I, et al. Guidelines for endobronchial ultrasound-transbronchial needle aspiration (EBUS-TBNA): Joint Indian Chest Society (ICS)/Indian Association for Bronchology (IAB) recommendations. Lung India. 2023;40(4):368–400.
9. Fernandes MGO, Santos VF, Martins N, Sucena MC, Passos MM, Marques MM, et al. Endobronchial ultrasound under moderate sedation versus general anesthesia. J Clin Med. 2018;7(11)
10. Casal RF, Lazarus DR, Kuhl K, Nogueras-Gonzalez G, Perusich S, Green LK, et al. Randomized trial of endobronchial ultrasound-guided transbronchial needle aspiration under general anesthesia versus moderate sedation. Am J Respir Crit Care Med. 2015;191(7):796–803.

6 Anesthesia for Robotic Bronchoscopy

John Pawlowski

6.1 Introduction

Robotic bronchoscopy (RB) or robotic-assisted bronchoscopy represents a recent technique to better sample lung lesions. Prior navigation techniques and visualization strategies have shown limitations in addressing smaller lesions and more peripheral lesions in the lung. Despite widespread screening, two-thirds of lung cancers are still identified in their late stages [1]. Other methods to sample peripheral lung lesions produce an incidence of pneumothorax of 20% and significant bleeding. Overall diagnostic yields from lung nodules using bronchoscopy are approximately 40% [2]. Thus, there have been concerted efforts to improve and develop better imaging, navigation, and sampling techniques to allow for better tissue diagnoses of lung tumors of small size, lower stage, and more peripheral location. In 2018, the FDA approved the first robotic-assisted bronchoscopy platform to address these needs.

At the time of this writing, there are three major robotic bronchoscopy (RB) systems in clinical use in the United States. While significant differences and potential advantages exist for each of the RB systems, this chapter will focus on their common features and clinical usefulness. Please refer to Diddams' article for a review, comparison, and discussion of these three RB systems [3]. Instead of a review of the contrasting features, this chapter will focus on the similarities, an explanation of how these features improve the precision and efficiency of lung tumor sampling, and how these RB systems might evolve in the future.

All the robotic-assisted systems have common advantages over the traditional trans-thoracic needle biopsy: lower pneumothorax rates, the ability to sample mediastinal nodes, and greater range in accessibility to biopsy. While flexible fiberoptic

J. Pawlowski (✉)
Department of Anesthesia, Critical Care and Pain Medicine, Beth Israel Deaconess Medical Center, Harvard Medical School, Boston, MA, USA
e-mail: jpawlows@bidmc.harvard.edu

M. Sarkiss (ed.), *Anesthesia for Interventional Pulmonary Procedures*,
https://doi.org/10.1007/978-3-032-12007-6_6

bronchoscopy is confined to the central lung locations, the smaller size of the robotic scope as well as the improved navigation systems allow RB to reach smaller airways in more peripheral regions. The development of radial bronchial ultrasound (rEBUS) does allow for more precision in locating lesions under 2 cm, but still poses difficulties in identifying the correct airways to transit [4].

Improvement in the navigation through airways came with the development of Super-Dimensional (Super-D) electromagnetic navigation bronchoscopy. This advance allows for tracking of the tip of the bronchoscope using an electromagnetic field generator. When paired with a recent computed tomography (CT) scan, the Super-D can provide an active location of the bronchoscope in the airway as well as a virtual representation of the target nodule.

While initial results of the Super-D system were promising, the multicentered trials and the long-term follow-up results are less optimistic. In the NAVIGATE trial, Folch et al. report an initial diagnostic yield for malignancy of 72.9%, with over half of the lesions being peripheral and with sizes less than 2 cm [5]. Follow-up results, however, found flaws with the Super-D systems. The positive predictive value in the NAVIGATE trial was 100%, yet the negative predictive value was only between 47% and 64%. In addition, other results from smaller volume centers showed less promising diagnostic yields. The technical difficulty of maintaining a precise stability during the periods of tissue sampling probably contributed to the worst results. Publication bias may also explain the earlier reported diagnostic successes. Reports that showed less favorable results for electromagnetic navigation and unresolved technical issues probably prompted the interest in the development of robotic-assisted bronchoscopy.

6.2 Robotic Bronchoscopy Procedure

Robotic platforms in both surgery and bronchoscopy offer better confined-space movement, ergonomics, and tremor suppression. While currently more costly, the robotic bronchoscopy devices may prove to bring better navigational features and more successful diagnostic yields [6]. With improved range of motion, robotic bronchoscopes can maneuver into more narrow and more tortuous airways than can conventional bronchoscopes. Omnidirectional movements and smaller external diameters make the airways more accessible to RB to the eighth bronchial division, rather than to the fourth division with standard bronchoscopy. Most RB systems utilize a navigational system using CT data or electromagnetic field data to maintain position. One system uses a proprietary shape-sensing system utilizing fiberoptic bend sensors to provide position data. Another system uses both electromagnetic navigations plus digital tomosynthesis guidance to establish orientation [3]. The purpose of all these navigation systems is to visualize the airway anatomy, the bronchoscope position, the target lesion in real-time three-dimensional overlapping images. In skilled hands, the navigational success rate of robotic bronchoscopy approaches 100% [7, 8]. The main advantage of the robotic bronchoscopy (RB) systems is their maneuverability to the target lesion. RB can get closer to the target lesion: within 9.4 mm versus 14.2 mm or 17.2 mm in Yarmus' study. The closer the proximity, the greater the chance of a central hit on the lesion during needle aspiration. In addition, RB provides better stabilization during needle biopsy compared to human hands (Figs. 6.1 and 6.2).

The complication rates for RB have been reported as lower than that of conventional transthoracic needle aspiration [9]. Both bleeding and pneumothorax rates were acceptable, and half of the pneumothorax patients did not require chest tube insertion. Another limitation of RB is the phenomenon of "CT-to-body divergence," defined as the difference between the static preprocedural CT image and the mobile lung during the procedure. In a recent report, the presence of CT-to-body divergence required repositioning of the bronchoscope in about 15% of the time and this repositioning negatively affected the diagnostic yield. With repositioning, the diagnostic yield dropped from 84% to 38% [10]. The causes for CT-to-body divergence are numerous and include absorptive atelectasis, mucous plugging, and pleural effusions. CT-to-body divergence is associated with procedural delays, excessive suctioning, excessive breath holds, RB learning curves, inadequate ventilation, and inadequate recruiting maneuvers. Thus, both underlying pathophysiologic and clinical performance conditions do influence the degree of CT-to-body divergence. Some of these clinical performance issues can be modified, and these issues form

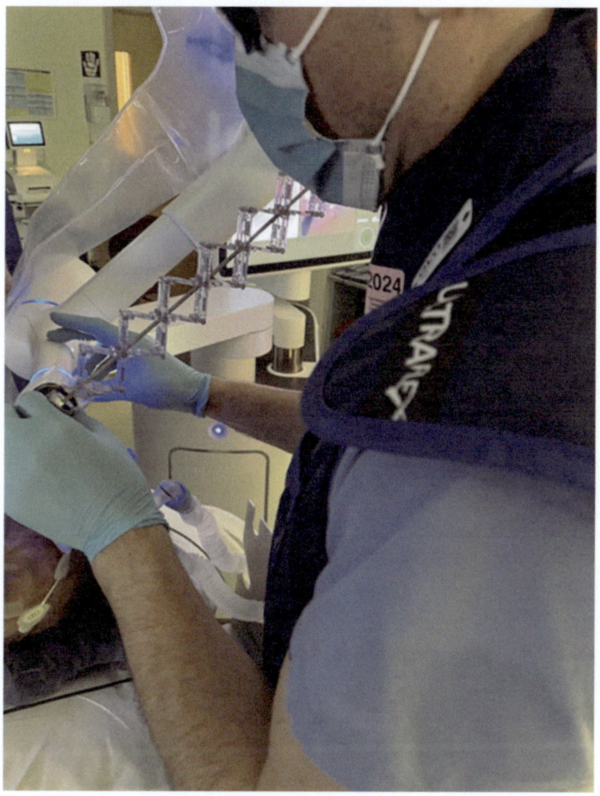

Fig. 6.1 Docking of the robotic bronchoscope through the endotracheal tube

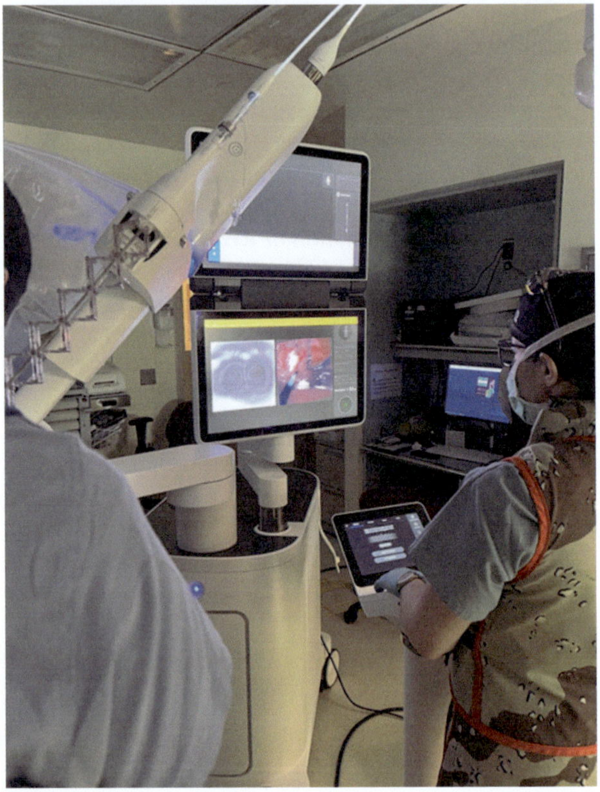

Fig. 6.2 Navigation through the airway

the basis of the anesthetic management presented later in this chapter. Not discussed in this chapter are the effects of histopathologic labeling, such as "nonspecific inflammation" or "nondiagnostic atypia" on the diagnostic yield. Case series now exist that show 100% tool-in-lesion using RB, yet only 86% diagnostic yield [11].

As mentioned previously, a key feature of robotic bronchoscopy is its stability and proximity to the target lesion. This stabile platform provides a potential opportunity for therapeutic treatments of lung cancers. Using a variety of energy types, tumors can be ablated laser, thermal, radiofrequency, microwave, and cryotherapy. In addition, chemotherapy drugs and immunotherapeutic agents can be used as local cancer treatment. RB can also be used to place fiducial markers in anticipation of surgical resection. Therefore, robotic bronchoscopy is poised to become an effective diagnostic and therapeutic strategy for lung cancer.

6.3 Anesthetic Strategies

While pulmonologists and anesthetists must share the same airway, they must also share the same mental models of safety, stability, and procedural success. To provide safety for the patient, sufficient oxygenation and ventilation must be provided.

Stability can refer to the normal vital signs throughout the procedure but can also refer to the need for reliable anatomy and freedom from excessive motion during the procedure. Procedural success also depends on the management of atelectasis, which can lead to obscurity of the target as well as increase the CT-to-body divergence.

The development of atelectasis from the provision of general anesthesia has long been recognized [12]. Occurring within minutes of induction, anesthesia-induced atelectasis can distort the lung anatomy and worsen divergence. Not visible by conventional fluoroscopy, the impact of atelectasis can be reliably detected using cone-beam computed tomography (CBCT). Casal et al. reported atelectasis in 40 percent of patients, which completely masked the lesion in 20% [13]. In a separate study, Sagar et al. noted atelectasis in 89% of patients and an association between atelectasis and increased body mass index (BMI) [14]. Patients in this study received general anesthesia, laryngeal mask airways (LMA), neuromuscular blocking agents (NMBs), an FiO2 of 100%, and little to no positive end-expiratory pressure (PEEP).

In practice, most anesthesia providers utilize general anesthesia for robotic bronchoscopy, but other techniques exist. One report by Bowling et al. compares the effects of general anesthesia versus intravenous (iv) sedation for electromagnetic navigation bronchoscopy [15]. These investigators report similar diagnostic yields, success rates, and complication rates in both groups. The only significant difference was the duration of the procedure, with the general anesthesia group lasting 58 minutes versus the IV sedation time of 43 minutes. Sedation consisted of a combination of fentanyl, midazolam, and propofol. No additional airway instrumentation was required in the IV sedation group. The complication rates were similar and did include three instances of pneumothorax, one of which required chest tube placement. This sedation group received deep sedation throughout the procedure. Another group (Minami, 2016) used only fentanyl and midazolam for sedation and averaged less than 50 mcg fentanyl and 2.5 mg midazolam for the entire bronchoscopic procedure. Fentanyl was given in 10 mcg increments and midazolam was given in 1 mg doses, suggesting light or at most moderate sedation. On a 5-point visual analog scale of discomfort, the patients averaged 2.02, indicating only mild discomfort and as proof, the authors noted that over 70% of these patients agreed to a subsequent bronchoscopy with the same sedation [16]. Therefore, both general anesthesia and sedation have been used successfully during bronchoscopic examination and diagnostic procedures. Both light and deep sedation have been employed. The choice of general anesthesia may be less based on patient comfort and more dependent control of ventilation.

With the use of general anesthesia comes the potential for therapeutic intervention using an endotracheal tube (ETT). The ETT allows the delivery of measured tidal volumes and accurate PEEP levels. With an ETT, recruiting maneuvers using vital capacity breaths and inspiratory holds can be accomplished. To accommodate the RB, usually an ETT of size 8.5 is used. Tidal volume settings are 8–10 cc per kilogram as tolerated. Due to the frequent disconnections to introduce pulmonary equipment and frequent requirements for suctioning, inhalational anesthetic concentrations may fluctuate unpredictably; so total intravenous anesthesia (TIVA) is preferred. Usually, propofol infusions of 150 mcg/kg/min and remifentanil infusions of 0.1 mcg/kg/min are employed with titration to the vital signs or to Bispectral index. To reduce diaphragmatic movement, NMBs such as rocuronium are used.

While conventional volume-controlled ventilation is most often used, several have advocated for jet ventilation as a mode to reduce the motion during electromagnetic navigation bronchoscopy [17]. These observations regarding the use of jet ventilation to reduce motion have been reported by other investigators such as those performing ablation techniques in cardiac electrophysiology units [18]. High-frequency jet ventilation, in particular, keeps tidal volumes very low: usually well below dead space. The low tidal volumes translate to small chest wall excursions. Jet ventilation does carry some additional risks of barotrauma and requires additional expertise by the anesthesia provider, which may limit the general acceptance of jet ventilation in RB procedures.

Preoperative assessment of patients scheduled for robotic bronchoscopy should include specific attention to risks for atelectasis. Patients should be screened for obesity and respiratory disease and should receive imaging to document pulmonary edema, pleural effusions, and atelectasis. Those with increased risk factors would probably benefit from preoperative incentive spirometry, but the timing and duration of this intervention are poorly characterized.

Preoxygenation during induction is a mainstay of anesthetic practice but may have negative effects on atelectasis, and, therefore, should be kept to a minimum. Complete denitrogenation from the use of 100% oxygen is well- described. Absorption atelectasis and alveolar collapse from the induction of anesthesia is only partially reversed by the use of postinduction recruiting maneuvers. Instead, an initial FiO2 of 0.6–0.8 was associated with minimal atelectasis on induction [19].

Any therapeutic use of electrocautery or laser during robotic bronchoscopy requires an FiO2 of 30% or less. Ideally, any use of thermal energy should be performed during a breath hold to reduce the chance of potential spread of the tissue destruction to distal areas.

The use of significant levels of positive end expiratory pressure (PEEP) is recommended to reduce the formation of atelectasis throughout the RB procedure [20]. Pritchett recommends 10–12 cm H2O of PEEP throughout the procedure, including during the times taken with breath holds. During these breath holds, the PEEP can be maintained using the adjustable pressure limiting (APL) valve in the manual mode of the anesthesia machine. In lower lobe biopsies and especially in obese patients, the PEEP levels may need to be higher. Use of high tidal volumes and high PEEP levels, however, should always be done with careful consideration for the possible hemodynamic changes such as decreased preload and decreased blood pressure.

The anesthesia provider needs to recognize the breathing circuit reflects a balance between the amount of fresh gas flow and the calculated leak from the APL valve. While one is adjusting the leak to maintain constant PEEP levels, one can also be affecting the filling of the ventilator bellows, for example. Care must be taken when switching between manual and automatic modes of ventilation to avoid periods of hypoventilation. Hypoventilation can lead to hypoxemia and can worsen atelectasis. The ventilator alarm may not be helpful as it tends to alarm continuously during disconnects and suctioning and, thus, may lead the provider to a state of alarm fatigue.

Assessment of the patient's readiness for extubation should follow full reversal of neuromuscular blockade and should be done with a full understanding of the patient's underlying respiratory status, comorbidities, and a respect for the deleterious effects of the procedure and the anesthetic on respiratory function. A train-of-four monitor with accelerometry should be used to gauge the adequacy of reversal. Spontaneous ventilation, adequate minute ventilation, tidal volume, and respiratory rate should be verified. Evidence of adequate oxygenation and ventilation should be present by SaO2 and CO2 monitors. Any signs of bronchospasm should be treated with bronchodilators; this author's practice is to give all patients bronchodilators at the conclusion of the procedure and prior to extubation. A postoperative chest X-ray in the recovery room to rule out pneumothorax is recommended.

6.4 Conclusion

Robotic bronchoscopy (RB) represents a novel series of technologies to better address the smaller and more peripheral lung lesions. RB includes navigational systems to identify the airway anatomy and visualize the target lesion. RB eliminates human fatigue and mitigates tremor to produce a more stable environment, for diagnostic tissue identification and, potentially, ablative therapy. The anesthetic techniques during RB are employed to minimize motion and maximize stability, while providing safe, pain-free, and hemodynamically normal conditions. A number of maneuvers to reduce the distorting effects of atelectasis have been mentioned. Some of these maneuvers include an increase in pressures and volumes in order to improve the anatomic visualization and confirm the tumor location. Care must be taken to limit these maneuvers to prevent barotrauma and volutrauma. With a close communication between the pulmonologist and the anesthesiologist, the patient will be able to have smaller lesions detected at earlier stages in their disease process, find definitive tissue diagnoses, and receive curative therapies in types of lung cancers that were, in previous times, found too late and when deemed inoperable.

References

1. Flores R. Association of stage shift and population mortality among patients with non-small cell lung cancer. JAMA Netw Open. 2021;4(12):e2137508.
2. Ost DE, Ernst A, Lei X, Kovitz KL, Benzaquen S, Diaz-Mendoza J, et al. Diagnostic yield and complications of bronchoscopy for peripheral lung lesions. Results of the AQuIRE registry. Am J Respir Crit Care Med. 2016;193(1):68–77.
3. Diddams MJ, Lee HJ. Robotic bronchoscopy: review of three systems. Life (Basel). 2023;13(2)
4. Becker H. Short history of the development of endobronchial ultrasound: a story of success. Clin Chest Ultrasound. 2009;37:128–39.

5. Folch EE, Pritchett MA, Nead MA, Bowling MR, Murgu SD, Krimsky WS, et al. Electromagnetic navigation bronchoscopy for peripheral pulmonary lesions: one-year results of the prospective, Multicenter NAVIGATE Study. J Thorac Oncol. 2019;14(3):445–58.
6. Chaddha U, Kovacs SP, Manley C, Hogarth DK, Cumbo-Nacheli G, Bhavani SV, et al. Robot-assisted bronchoscopy for pulmonary lesion diagnosis: results from the initial multicenter experience. BMC Pulm Med. 2019;19(1):243.
7. Yarmus L, Akulian J, Wahidi M, Chen A, Steltz JP, Solomon SL, et al. A prospective randomized comparative study of three guided Bronchoscopic approaches for investigating pulmonary nodules: the PRECISION-1 study. Chest. 2020;157(3):694–701.
8. Khan F, Seaman J, Hunter TD, Ribeiro D, Laxmanan B, Kalsekar I, et al. Diagnostic outcomes of robotic-assisted bronchoscopy for pulmonary lesions in a real-world multicenter community setting. BMC Pulm Med. 2023;23(1):161.
9. Yu Lee-Mateus A, Reisenauer J, Garcia-Saucedo JC, Abia-Trujillo D, Buckarma EH, Edell ES, et al. Robotic-assisted bronchoscopy versus CT-guided transthoracic biopsy for diagnosis of pulmonary nodules. Respirology. 2023;28(1):66–73.
10. Agrawal A, Ho E, Chaddha U, Demirkol B, Bhavani SV, Hogarth DK, et al. Factors associated with diagnostic accuracy of robotic bronchoscopy with 12-month follow-up. Ann Thorac Surg. 2023;115(6):1361–8.
11. Benn BS, Romero AO, Lum M, Krishna G. Robotic-assisted navigation bronchoscopy as a paradigm shift in peripheral lung access. Lung. 2021;199(2):177–86.
12. Brismar B, Hedenstierna G, Lundquist H, Strandberg A, Svensson L, Tokics L. Pulmonary densities during anesthesia with muscular relaxation--a proposal of atelectasis. Anesthesiology. 1985;62(4):422–8.
13. Casal RF, Sarkiss M, Jones AK, Stewart J, Tam A, Grosu HB, et al. Cone beam computed tomography-guided thin/ultrathin bronchoscopy for diagnosis of peripheral lung nodules: a prospective pilot study. J Thorac Dis. 2018;10(12):6950–9.
14. Sagar AS, Sabath BF, Eapen GA, Song J, Marcoux M, Sarkiss M, et al. Incidence and location of atelectasis developed during bronchoscopy under general anesthesia: the I-LOCATE trial. Chest. 2020;158(6):2658–66.
15. Bowling MR, Kohan MW, Walker P, Efird J, Ben OS. The effect of general anesthesia versus intravenous sedation on diagnostic yield and success in electromagnetic navigation bronchoscopy. J Bronchology Interv Pulmonol. 2015;22(1):5–13.
16. Minami D, Takigawa N, Watanabe H, Ninomiya T, Kubo T, Ohashi K, et al. Safety and discomfort during bronchoscopy performed under sedation with fentanyl and midazolam: a prospective study. Jpn J Clin Oncol. 2016;46(9):871–4.
17. Webb TN, Bonta DV, Masters R, Parks C, Bechara R. Jet ventilation decreases target motion and increases yield of ENB especially in lesions with negative bronchus sign. J Bronchol Interv Pulmonol. 2020;27(1):14–21.
18. Elkassabany N, Garcia F, Tschabrunn C, Raiten J, Gao W, Chaichana K, et al. Anesthetic management of patients undergoing pulmonary vein isolation for treatment of atrial fibrillation using high-frequency jet ventilation. J Cardiothorac Vasc Anesth. 2012;26(3):433–8.
19. Edmark L, Kostova-Aherdan K, Enlund M, Hedenstierna G. Optimal oxygen concentration during induction of general anesthesia. Anesthesiology. 2003;98(1):28–33.
20. Pritchett MA, Lau K, Skibo S, Phillips KA, Bhadra K. Anesthesia considerations to reduce motion and atelectasis during advanced guided bronchoscopy. BMC Pulm Med. 2021;21(1):240.

Anesthesia for Patients with Central Airway Obstruction

7

Mi Wang and Andrew Zura

7.1 Introduction

Central airway obstruction (CAO) is defined as the occlusion of >50% of the trachea, mainstem bronchi, bronchus intermedius, or lobar bronchus [1]. A wide variety of disease processes can cause CAO (Table 7.1). The most common cause of malignant CAO is direct extension from an adjacent tumor—usually bronchogenic, followed by esophageal and thyroid carcinoma. The most common nonmalignant CAO is postintubation or post-tracheostomy injury [2].

Table 7.1 Etiologies of central airway obstruction

Benign	Malignant
Foreign body	Primary carcinoma
Excessive dynamic airway collapse (EDAC)	Metastatic carcinoma
Tracheomalacia	Tumor invasion from
Benign tumors	Larynx
Papillomatosis	Esophagus
Stenosis related to trauma or inflammatory process	Mediastinum
	Lymphoma

M. Wang
Department of Anesthesiology and Perioperative Medicine, The University of Texas MD Anderson Cancer Center, Houston, TX, USA

A. Zura (✉)
Anesthesiology Institute, Cleveland Clinic Foundation, Cleveland, OH, USA
e-mail: zuraa@ccf.org

M. Sarkiss (ed.), *Anesthesia for Interventional Pulmonary Procedures*,
https://doi.org/10.1007/978-3-032-12007-6_7

7.2 Initial Evaluation

The factors influencing each patient's unique presentation are complex, including the underlying disease, the location and acuity of obstruction, and overall health status. Respiratory symptoms develop when the obstruction decreases airflow to a critical threshold. The air hunger sensation frequently reported by these patients is usually related to a perceived increased work of breathing and not hypoxia or hypercapnia. The literature has widely cited that once the endoluminal diameter of the trachea is decreased to less than 8 mm (exertional) or 5 mm (at rest) symptoms will develop [2, 3]. However, such fixed numbers have been questioned. Besides the narrowed endoluminal diameter, other flow limitation variables exist, such as length and the pressure gradient across the obstruction [4].

7.2.1 Radiographic Evaluation

Plain chest X-rays rarely provide significant information. They cannot determine airway invasion or aid in procedure planning [5]. Chest X-rays can identify obvious pathology, such as tracheal deviation. Baseline chest X-rays can also provide rapid postintervention comparisons as it is often impractical to obtain serial CT scans.

CT has been recognized as the imaging modality of choice. It can investigate the location, length, maximal degree of obstruction, and the relationship to surrounding structures. In recent years, multidetector CT (MDCT) imaging and various three-dimensional imaging techniques have become more readily available [6]. Extraluminal 3-D reconstruction allows for a more anatomically relevant evaluation of the airways concerning surrounding structures, while intraluminal 3-D reconstruction allows for a virtual bronchoscopic evaluation [7]. CT can also document dynamic airway collapse [8].

7.2.2 Pulmonary Function Test

One of three basic patterns of the flow-volume loop are observed in patients with central airway obstruction during PFTs (Fig. 7.1). A fixed obstruction, such as tracheal stenosis, will limit airflow in both inspiration and expiration, whether the lesion is intrathoracic or extrathoracic. In variable obstruction, the impact on airflow varies depending on the relative pressure differences between the airway lumen and surrounding tissue. Variable obstruction is often seen with a flexible or floppy lesion, such as ECAC. The airway tends to collapse during expiration if the flexible lesion is intrathoracic [9].

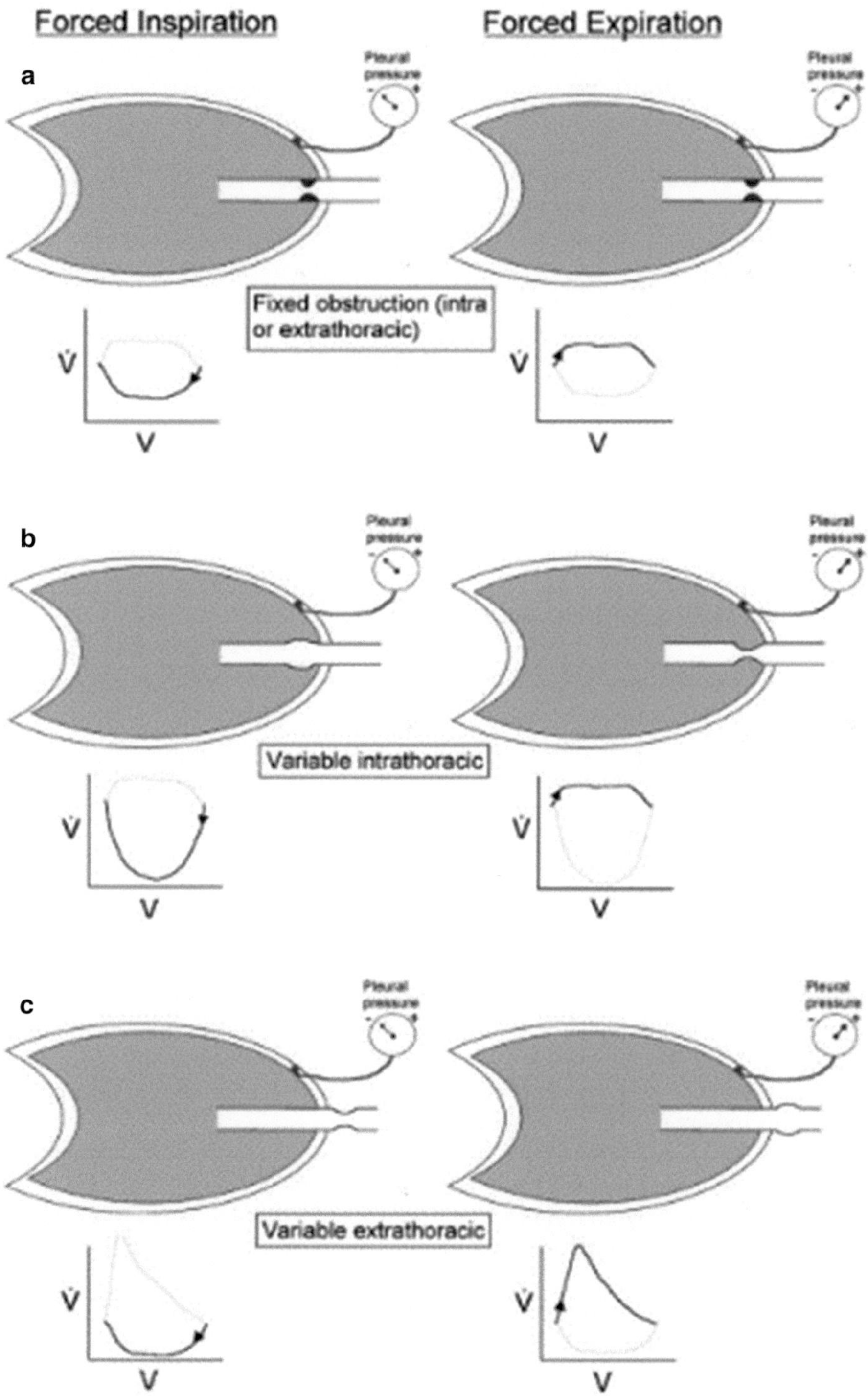

Fig. 7.1 Flow volume loops for patients with central airway obstruction. (**a**) Fixed intra- or extrathoracic obstruction, (**b**) variable intrathoracic obstruction, and (**c**) variable extrathoracic obstruction. (Needs copyright permission from [9])

Table 7.2 Types of interventional bronchoscopic procedures

Diagnostic bronchoscopy	Advanced diagnostic bronchoscopy	Therapeutic bronchoscopy
Bronchoalveolar lavage (BAL) Endobronchial biopsy Transbronchial biopsy (TBBX) Brushing Transbronchial needle aspiration (TBNA) Flexible bronchoscopy airway exam	Linear endobronchial ultrasound transbronchial needle aspiration (EBUS-TBNA) Radial endobronchial ultrasound (rEBUS) Electromagnetic navigation (EMN) Cryobiopsy	*Rigid bronchoscopy with ablative techniques* Argon plasma coagulation (APC) Electrocautery Cryoablation Spray cryotherapy Photodynamic therapy (PDT) Laser *Rigid bronchoscopy with stent placement* Metallic stents Silicon stent *Rigid bronchoscopy with tumor debulking* Microdebriment Coring

7.3 Bronchoscopic Procedures for CAO

The role of interventional pulmonology in managing CAO is continually expanding [10, 11]. The advancement of devices, including laser probes, stents, cryoprobes, argon plasma coagulation, inflatable balloons, and ultrasound probes, has benefited patients with increased diagnostic and therapeutic applications [12]. Different procedures require different anesthetic management based on the complexity of the procedure and coexisting patient factors (Table 7.2) [13].

7.4 Anesthesia Strategies

The American College of Chest Physicians recommends all patients undergoing bronchoscopy receive topical anesthesia, analgesia, and sedation as it improves patient tolerance and satisfaction [14]. Basic diagnostic bronchoscopy procedures can be performed under minimal sedation. Advanced diagnostic and therapeutic procedures require a deeper level of anesthesia.

Topical anesthesia blunts the airway response to procedural stimulation, decreases cough, and reduces the required dose of sedatives [14]. For clinicians who utilize the spray-as-you-go technique, 1% lidocaine has been found to significantly lower the total dose required while achieving the same efficacy compared to 2% lidocaine [15].

There is currently no consensus regarding the best technique to achieve deeper levels of sedation. Various sedation protocols using midazolam, propofol, dexmedetomidine, or ketamine have also showed promising results [16–19].

Total intravenous anesthesia (TIVA) using propofol infusions is commonly used for advanced diagnostic and therapeutic bronchoscopy. It can be used for both sedation and general anesthesia. The propofol dosing reported consists of an initial bolus of 0.5–1.0 mg.kg^{-1} followed by infusion ranging from 75 mcg.kg^{-1}.min^{-1} to 250 mcg.kg^{-1}.min^{-1} [13, 20]. Propofol titration is guided by the desired anesthesia depth and the patient's hemodynamics. Electroencephalographic methods (e.g., BIS) can aid monitoring but are not mandatory [21].

Volatile anesthetic agents are generally not recommended as the integrity of the ventilatory circuit is frequently interrupted, causing pollution of the procedure room and inadequate delivery of the agent to anesthetize the patient [22–24]. The beneficial effect of intravenous corticosteroids in reducing the incidence of post-bronchoscopy laryngeal edema is lacking evidence [25]. The routine use of anticholinergic also fails to demonstrate a general clinical benefit [14].

7.5 Ventilation and Airway Strategies

Ventilation is challenging for symptomatic CAO patients for multiple reasons [26, 27]. The patient's central airway is already compromised. Endoscopic instrumentation further occludes the lumen. Intervention-related complications, like bleeding and clots, can further worsen the obstruction.

Ventilation and airway strategies range from spontaneous ventilation without an airway device under minimal sedation to positive-pressure ventilation under general anesthesia. They are determined by the patient's underlying disease, comorbidities, and the desired procedural condition [22, 28]. The most common initial airways are an orotracheal tube, a supraglottic airway device, or a rigid bronchoscope [27]. During the procedure, the initial airway is changed to another device due to a need for improved operating conditions. For example, a rigid bronchoscope can be changed to an ETT for more definitive airway control [27].

Different underlying pathologies of CAO dictate different challenges. Malignant or nonmalignant tracheal stenosis has similar ventilation profiles, with fixed airflow limitation during inspiration and expiration. This contrasts with dynamic obstruction, for example, tracheomalacia, whose flow limit occurs during expiration with the inspiration phase intact [29]. Probably the most feared complication is the extremely rare but reported fatal airway collapse related to massive anterior mediastinal mass, which can have both the features of fixed and dynamic airway obstructions [30]. The following discussion will include the abovementioned three categories to highlight their different challenges.

7.6 Anterior Mediastinal Mass

Mediastinal tumors are uncommon and represent 3% of tumors seen within the chest. Most of them occur in the anterior compartment, which includes a wide variety of benign and malignant tumors afflicting patients of all ages [31] (Table 7.3).

Table 7.3 Anterior mediastinal compartment boundaries, contents, and etiology of anterior mediastinal tumors [32, 33]

Anterior mediastinum boundaries	Anterior: sternum Posterior: pericardium Superior: thoracic inlet Inferior: diaphragm
Anterior mediastinal contents	Lymph nodes Thymus gland Thyroid gland extension Fat Nerves Vessels
Anterior mediastina tumors	Lymphadenopathy Lymphoma Thymic tumor (benign/malignant) Thyroid mass (benign/malignant) Parathyroid mass (benign/malignant) Lipoma Paraganglioma Germ cell tumors

The most common anterior mediastinal masses are thymic malignancy, lymphoma, and thyroid tumors [34, 35].

Symptoms are seen in 60% of these patients during their initial evaluation [36]. They can be categorized into two groups. (1) Result of direct compression and/or invasion of surrounding structures (2) Paraneoplastic syndromes associated with tumor-secreting hormones, antibodies, and cytokines.

The most common symptom is cough. Moderate cardiopulmonary symptoms included dyspnea on exertion, chest pain, fatigue, and vocal cord paralysis. Severe cardiorespiratory findings were defined as orthopnea, stridor, cyanosis, jugular vein distension, or superior vena cava syndrome [37]. Bechard found that the occurrence of cardiorespiratory signs and symptoms at the initial presentation was correlated with perioperative complications [38].

Any airway compression-related symptoms prompt further thorough evaluation. The most dreaded respiratory decompensation is caused by mechanical compression of the trachea, main bronchi, or both by the tumor. Orthopnea is a big warning sign. Some experts grade the airway compression-related symptoms depending on how well the patient can tolerate the supine position.

Asymptomatic: patient can lie supine without symptoms.
Mild: patient can lie supine with some cough/pressure sensation.
Moderate: patient can lie supine for only short periods.
Severe: patient cannot tolerate supine position.

There may be several reasons why changing to a supine position precipitates airway collapse [30].

Anterior mediastinal mass lying on top of vital structures and compressing them compared to sitting position where there is less impact.

The supine position makes the tight mediastinal compartment tighter, secondary to a reduction in the transverse diameter of the thorax and a cephalad displacement of the diaphragm. As the central blood volume increases, the size and weight of well-vascularized mediastinal tumors considerably increase.

One should perform a postural symptoms physical exam in these patients. Often, symptomatic patients report feeling better with sitting/semi-sitting positions. If these favorable positions are determined preoperatively, repositioning the patient could facilitate rescuing patients from tumor compression intraoperatively.

Chest X-rays, CTs, and bronchoscopy are routinely utilized in the workup of CAO. Detecting any compression or encroachment of the heart and major vessels is important. If the patient has SVC syndrome or other symptoms, for example, orthopnea, cyanosis, jugular distension further cardiac workup, including TTE or TEE, is warranted. If feasible, TTE or TEE should be performed in different positions.

Clinical investigators have presented models for preoperative risk to stratify patients better and predict outcomes. Bechard et al. reported results from a retrospective study of 98 patients (105 anesthetic cases). Complications occurred in 14.3% (15/105) of cases. Risk factors for perioperative complications included the presence of a pericardial effusion; tracheal compression >50%; a combined restrictive/obstructive pulmonary defect; and cardiorespiratory symptoms on initial presentation [38]. A study of 117 pediatric patients (median age 14.1 years) with mediastinal masses undergoing a mix of anesthetic types reported an anesthetic complication rate of 9.4% (11/117 cases). In that trial, compression of the mainstem bronchus or great vessels, orthopnea, and upper body edema were strongly predictive for perioperative complications [39].

7.6.1 Anesthesia Management

Frequent procedures related to mediastinal masses include interventional bronchoscopy, mediastinoscopy, sternotomy, thoracotomy, and thoracoscopic biopsy. For patients deemed exceptionally high risk of cardiopulmonary collapse, the options tend to be either an awake procedure with local anesthesia or mechanical circulatory support with or without general anesthesia. An awake percutaneous needle biopsy guided by CT, MRI, or ultrasound is widely used as a useful alternative to thoracotomy and mediastinoscopy [40–42]. Mechanical circulatory support has been reported in the literature for large mediastinal mass patients deemed exceptionally high risk of cardiopulmonary collapse [43]. Its value and effectiveness is questionable [44]. Even with a primed pump and a prepared team, cannulating and establishing adequate circulation is time-consuming [45]. Some experts suggested guidewire or cannula placement before anesthetic induction to facilitate the rapid institution of mechanical circulatory support should the need arise [46, 47]. Others believed that even a guidewire or cannula in place might not be adequate in emergent situations once hemodynamic collapse occurs. They advocated for the institution of mechanical circulatory support before anesthetic induction for extremely symptomatic high-risk patients [44, 48].

Most of the procedures we encounter at the bronchoscopy suites fall between the abovementioned options. General anesthesia is indicated since the patients cannot tolerate being awake, and ECMO is not feasible. There is no consensus on the best practice for conducting general anesthesia.

The traditional recommendation is that maintaining spontaneous breathing is safer and preserves airway patency compared to positive pressure ventilation (PPV) with or without paralysis. This classic teaching has been passed on for decades, with the earliest case reports dating back to the 1970s; however, there is a lack of evidence to support its value.

Within the last two decades, case reports of intraoperative fatalities have become exceedingly rare. New literature has shown that positive-pressure ventilation and neuromuscular blockade are well tolerated [33, 49, 50]. Between January 1994 and July 2000, 105 anesthetic cases were performed on 98 adult patients with mediastinal masses in a tertiary university hospital. General anesthesia was selected in 97 of the cases with 79 receiving neuromuscular blockade at induction. No cases of airway collapse occurred [38]. In another case series of 57 adult patients with anterior mediastinal masses getting general anesthesia, 90% received neuromuscular blockade during induction, and 100% received neuromuscular blockade during maintenance without any incident [50].

In 2018, Hartigan reported bronchoscopic observation during a staged anesthesia induction in a large anterior mediastinal mass patient [51]. This case report is considered ground-breaking as it provided direct and objective evidence that there was little change in airway patency between awake spontaneous ventilation and anesthetized PPV with or without muscle paralysis. His team further validated their findings with a prospective single-center observational study [52]. Four ventilatory stages were studied in 17 patients with anterior mediastinal masses: awake spontaneous ventilation, anesthetized spontaneous ventilation, anesthetized positive pressure ventilation, and anesthetized positive pressure ventilation after muscle paralysis. The authors found that (I) induction of general anesthesia, PPV, or the addition of muscle paralysis did not decrease the anteroposterior compressed airway diameter. (II) There was a reported visual subjective improvement in airway patency with the institution of PPV that persisted and further improved after muscle paralysis [52].

The key to successful PPV is to prevent air trapping by mimicking the spontaneous ventilation volume, respiratory rate, and I:E ratio to recreate the prolonged expiration in awake spontaneously ventilating patients and allow for complete exhalation of the inspired tidal volume through the narrowed airway. If the air trapping during PPV is not recognized, the accumulated high intrathoracic pressure can diminish venous return precipitating hemodynamic collapse not only by decreasing cardiac output but also by worsening the mechanical tumor compression on the heart. Fiorelli did an observational study using noninvasive positive pressure ventilation (NIPPV) as a surrogate for self-expanding stents for symptomatic relief in severe tracheal stenosis patients with large mediastinal mass [53]. They measured the peak inspiratory flow (PIF) and peak expiratory flow (PEF) after adding PEEP of 10 cmH2O through a face mask while supine and spontaneously breathing. Out of 13 patients, 11 improved in both PIF and PEF. The other two patients had no significant improvement with PEEP and were deemed not suitable for palliative stents.

Since induction of general anesthesia in the supine position can exacerbate mediastinal mass compression due to decreased FRC and thoracic volume, Sarkiss et al. published a stepwise induction of general anesthesia and a transition to positive pressure ventilation and muscle relaxation that functions as their protocol for rigid bronchoscopy for airway stenting in patients with central airway obstruction at MD Anderson Cancer Center [54].

I. Slow intravenous induction with propofol infusion in a semi-sitting position to avoid acute hemodynamic changes associated with administering a propofol bolus.
II. Continuous measurement of the tidal volume and airway pressure during induction by applying the anesthesia circuit's face mask to the patient to monitor for adequate air exchange.
III. Muscle relaxation and positive pressure ventilation with an I:E ratio of 1:4 and low respiratory rate to avoid air trapping.
IV. Insertion of the rigid bronchoscope past the obstruction area to stent the airway open and relief any air trapping during the anesthesia induction.
V. In the event of hemodynamic compromise secondary to air trapping and the inability to pass the rigid bronchoscope past the obstruction, passing the flexible bronchoscope past the obstruction and applying suctioning can relieve the air trapping and lung hyperinflation with restoration of the hemodynamics.

Due to the rarity of the patient population, prospective randomized controlled studies are lacking. Over the last few decades, anesthesia management of mediastinal mass procedures has evolved from opinion-based explanations in case reports or series to direct visualization and measurement of airway dynamics in observational studies. Further studies are needed to establish best practice recommendations.

7.7 Expiratory Central Airway Collapse (ECAC)

Usually, the central airway's cross-sectional area (CSA) increases during inspiration and decreases during expiration, secondary to physiologic transthoracic pressure changes. This dynamic expiratory central airway narrowing can become pathologically excessive and cause clinical symptoms, termed expiratory central airway collapse (ECAC). ECAC includes two distinct entities: tracheobronchomalacia (TBM) and excessive dynamic airway collapse (EDAC).

TBM results from pathologic softening of the cartilaginous tracheal or mainstem bronchial rings and is well established in the literature. EDAC, to the contrary, is associated with a degenerating posterior membrane while the anterior cartilaginous rings are intact. The definition of EDAC is simply a more than 50% reduction in CSA from the bulging of the posterior membrane during the expiration [55]. The imaging diagnosis does not necessarily correlate with the clinical findings. Boiselle found that 78% of healthy subjects with normal PFTs met the criteria of EDAC. Some had CSA reductions as much as 80–90% [56] . Chronic pulmonary diseases are frequently associated with ECAC, with the worst TBM among morbidly obese COPD patients [57, 58]. In asthmatic patients, EDAC is much more frequently observed than TBM. Other factors reportedly associated with both TBM and EDAC are related to age and female sex [59] (Fig. 7.2).

The symptoms of ECAC are often challenging to differentiate from those of COPD or asthma. You can often see dyspnea refractory to bronchodilator treatment or disproportionate to PFT results, unexplained paroxysmal dyspnea, recurrent COPD or asthma exacerbations, chronic cough, especially with sputum retention or "seal barking" sound [60, 61].

ECAC can be confirmed by paired inspiratory-dynamic expiratory chest CT [8, 62]. Dynamic flexible bronchoscopy using minimal sedation is considered the "gold standard" with high inter- and intraobserver agreements [63]. PFTs are often relatively normal without any other pulmonary disease. There is no specific finding in pulmonary studies that is diagnostic of ECAC. For patients with severe symptoms matching the imaging and bronchoscopic findings, treatments include noninvasive positive-pressure ventilation, bronchoscopic stent insertion, and surgical tracheobronchoplasty [55, 64]. Most patients report an improved quality of life after tracheobronchoplasty [65].

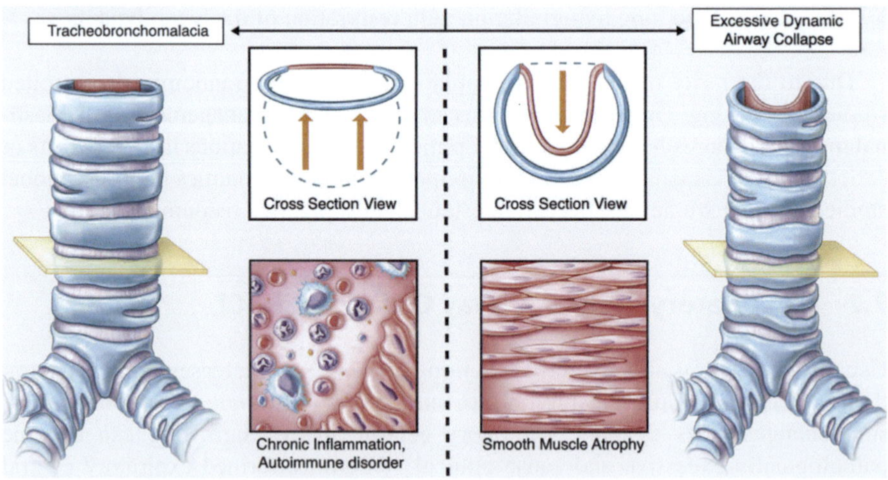

Fig. 7.2 Etiology, anatomical, and flow changes associated with expiratory central airway collapse (ECAC). (Need copyright permission from PMID: 30279064)

7.7.1 Anesthesia Management Related to ECAC in Bronchoscopy Suite

The most common procedure relating to ECAC in the bronchoscopy suite is the awake flexible bronchoscopy to confirm the diagnosis of EDAC. After adequate topical anesthesia, the patient is directed to inhale and exhale forcefully. Simultaneously, the degree of collapse of the tracheobronchial tree is evaluated by direct visualization through a bronchoscope at six different levels: cricoid, mid trachea, distal trachea, proximal left mainstem, proximal right mainstem, and proximal bronchus intermedius. The expiratory dynamic collapse is graded based on visual estimation. Degree of collapse is defined as mild (70–79%), moderate (80–89%), and severe (> 90%) [55, 64]. If the collapse is significant, a titrated CPAP trial is conducted to determine sufficient positive pressure to maintain airway patency.

Unexpected significant airway obstruction due to ECAC perioperatively is rare and probably underrecognized. Only a handful of case reports are found in the literature [66–70]. The intraoperative interventions in these case reports can be summarized as (1) physical stenting by single- or double-lumen endotracheal tubes, (2) PEEP serving as pneumatic stenting, and (3) resuming spontaneous ventilation and waking the patients. All ECAC symptoms were reversible except for the case reported by Lyaker [71]. In their report, the patient with BMI 62 failed extubation multiple times in the ICU postoperatively. EDAC might play a role in acute-on-chronic refractory respiratory failure, but it is unlikely the sole cause.

In summary, ECAC can cause significant unexpected obstruction during anesthesia in patients without a previous diagnosis. Unlike the nondynamic obstructions, for example, kinked ETT, mucus plug, or PTX, ECAC manifests sudden increased airway resistance or abnormal ETCO2 tracing, mainly in the expiratory phase. The threshold for a bronchoscopic exam should be low when suspecting ECAC. If no obstruction is observed from the exam, then bronchospasm might be the cause. If ECAC is suggested, other than physical and pneumatic stenting of the obstruction and resuming spontaneous respiration, other interventions, including jet ventilation or helium-oxygen, have been suggested [55, 64]. In extreme cases, ECMO can be considered when effective ventilation cannot be restored. An algorithm is provided to guide the management of a suspected ECAC [55] (Fig. 7.3).

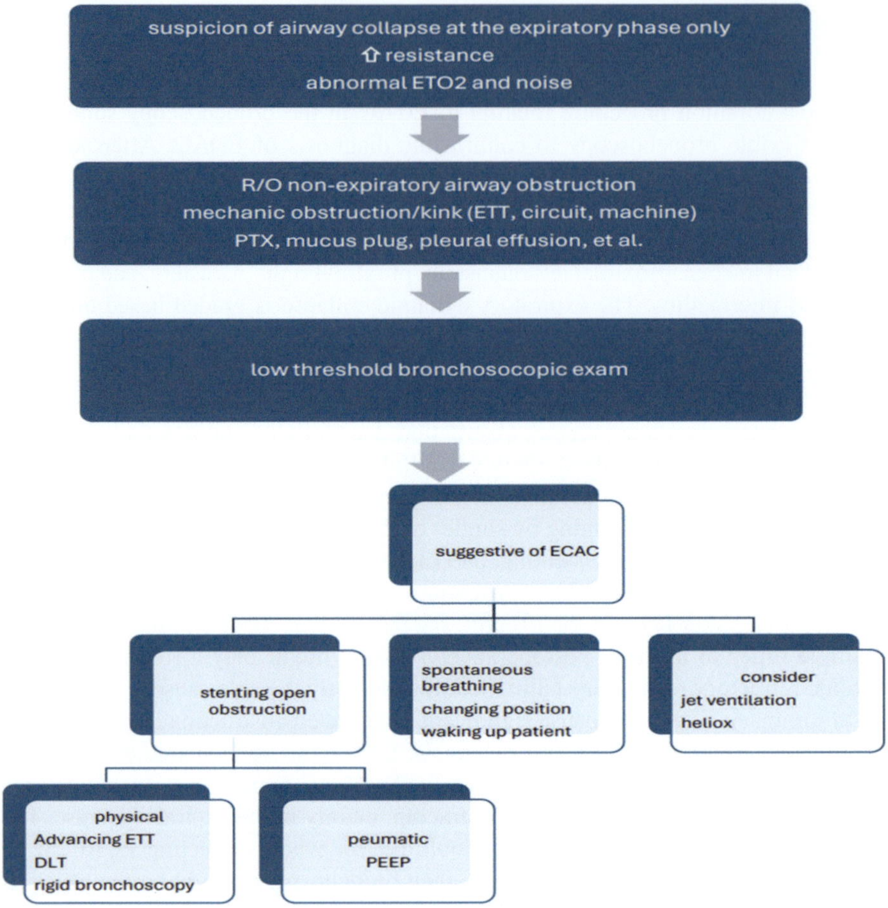

Fig. 7.3 Algorithm for the management of patients with suspected expiratory central airway collapse

7.8 Laryngotracheal Stenosis

Both malignant and benign disease processes can cause laryngotracheal stenosis (LTS). The resultant central airway obstruction affects both inspiration and expiration compared to the dynamic obstruction, mainly at expiration, of patients with ECAC. The common underlying pathologies include postintubation injury from ETT or tracheostomy idiopathic subglottic stenosis, tumors. Other causes of LTS can be related infections, GERD, or surgical scarring.

Surgical resection is the definitive treatment for severe tracheal stenosis. Factors such as severe comorbidities, length, and location of the stricture can preclude patients from undergoing curative surgery. Interventional bronchoscopy plays an essential role in treating LTS. Dilation, electrosurgery, micro debridement, airway stenting, and pharmacological treatment with mitomycin C and intralesional steroid injection are options.

7.8.1 Anesthetic Management

Patients presenting with stridor warrant immediate clinical attention as an ominous sign of close to complete airway obstruction. The office endoscopic exam by ENT team as well as CT scan provides valuable information. If there is concern that the stenotic airway might not be sufficient to permit general anesthesia induction, awake intubation, awake tracheostomy, or ECMO can be considered.

IV induction of general anesthesia, including muscle paralysis and maintained with TIVA, is commonly practiced. Propofol alone or in conjunction with a remifentanil infusion is titrated to the desired effect. If rigid bronchoscopy is indicated, dexamethasone during induction is often used to decrease airway edema postoperatively. Muscle relaxation facilitates instrumentation and minimizes the iatrogenic injury from the patient's cough or movement during rigid bronchoscopy. Suggamadex is frequently used to reverse muscle paralysis at the end of the procedure.

Intraoperative ventilation strategies vary depending on the procedures and the severity of the patient's tracheal stenosis. In a study by Zhu [72], ventilation strategies for patients undergoing urgent tracheal stenting were based on the location and etiology of tracheal stenosis. For postintubation tracheal stenosis, where the stenosis is the upper third of the trachea LMAs were used. For the tracheal tumors located in the middle of the trachea in patients who cannot tolerate conventional intubation, veno-arterial ECMO was used successfully. For the tumors located in the lower third of the trachea, a cuffed tracheal tube was used. Low-frequency jet ventilation in rigid bronchoscopy was used in the stenosis located in the right or left main bronchus.

For immediate postoperative severe stridor, pharmacological treatment aimed at decreasing the airway edema includes nebulized racemic epinephrine and IV dexamethasone, whose effect on adult airway edema prevention is controversial [73]. Heliox, a mixture of helium (70%) and oxygen (30%), delivered using a nonrebreathing face mask at 10 L/min can be very useful in these situations [74]. The authors have used heliox as the carrier gas to nebulize racemic epinephrine in an extremely stenotic patient whose stridor was refractory to routine treatments. Heliox can often be weaned off after several hours, and the emergent reintubation or surgical airway can be avoided.

References

1. Ost DE, Ernst A, Grosu HB, Lei X, Diaz-Mendoza J, Slade M, et al. Therapeutic bronchoscopy for malignant central airway obstruction: success rates and impact on dyspnea and quality of life. Chest. 2015;147(5):1282–98.
2. Ernst A, Feller-Kopman D, Becker HD, Mehta AC. Central airway obstruction. Am J Respir Crit Care Med. 2004;169(12):1278–97.
3. Wahidi MM, Herth FJ, Ernst A. State of the art: interventional pulmonology. Chest. 2007;131(1):261–74.
4. Mudambi L, Miller R, Eapen GA. Malignant central airway obstruction. J Thorac Dis. 2017;9(Suppl 10):S1087–S110.
5. Le-Khac B, Nguyen-Dang K, Vu-Hoai N, Nguyen-Thanh N, Duong-Minh N, Tran-Ngoc TH, et al. Challenges in diagnosis and management of central airway obstruction: case series. SAGE Open Med Case Rep. 2024;12:2050313X231225327.
6. Ozgul MA, Ozgul G, Cetinkaya E, Abul Y, Kirkil G, Seyhan EC, et al. Multiplanar and two-dimensional imaging of central airway stenting with multidetector computed tomography. Multidiscip Respir Med. 2012;7(1):27.
7. Natale G, Leonardi B, Messina G, Bergameo G, Di Filippo V, Chisari G, et al. Three-dimensional lung reconstructions for the localization of lung nodules to be resected during surgery. Thorac Cancer. 2023;14(34):3389–96.
8. Baroni RH, Feller-Kopman D, Nishino M, Hatabu H, Loring SH, Ernst A, et al. Tracheobronchomalacia: comparison between end-expiratory and dynamic expiratory CT for evaluation of central airway collapse. Radiology. 2005;235(2):635–41.
9. Hayes D Jr, Kraman SS. The physiologic basis of spirometry. Respir Care. 2009;54(12):1717–26.
10. Shafiq M, Lee H, Yarmus L, Feller-Kopman D. Recent advances in interventional pulmonology. Ann Am Thorac Soc. 2019;16(7):786–96.
11. Hsia D, Musani AI. Interventional pulmonology. Med Clin North Am. 2011;95(6):1095–114.
12. Arias S, Lee HJ. The future of interventional pulmonology. Semin Respir Crit Care Med. 2014;35(6):763–8.
13. de Lima A, Kheir F, Majid A, Pawlowski J. Anesthesia for interventional pulmonology procedures: a review of advanced diagnostic and therapeutic bronchoscopy. Can J Anaesth. 2018;65(7):822–36.
14. Wahidi MM, Jain P, Jantz M, Lee P, Mackensen GB, Barbour SY, et al. American College of Chest Physicians consensus statement on the use of topical anesthesia, analgesia, and sedation during flexible bronchoscopy in adult patients. Chest. 2011;140(5):1342–50.
15. Kaur H, Dhooria S, Aggarwal AN, Gupta D, Behera D, Agarwal R. A randomized trial of 1% vs 2% lignocaine by the spray-as-you-go technique for topical anesthesia during flexible bronchoscopy. Chest. 2015;148(3):739–45.
16. Dreher M, Ekkernkamp E, Storre JH, Kabitz HJ, Windisch W. Sedation during flexible bronchoscopy in patients with pre-existing respiratory failure: Midazolam versus Midazolam plus Alfentanil. Respiration. 2010;79(4):307–14.
17. Muller T, Thummel K, Cornelissen CG, Kruger S, Dreher M. Analogosedation during flexible bronchoscopy using a combination of midazolam, propofol and fentanyl - a retrospective analysis. PLoS One. 2017;12(4):e0175394.
18. Wu SH, Lu DV, Hsu CD, Lu IC. The effectiveness of low-dose dexmedetomidine infusion in sedative flexible bronchoscopy: a retrospective analysis. Medicina (Kaunas). 2020;56(4)
19. Fruchter O, Manevich Y, Carmi U, Rozengarten D, Kramer MR. Prospective randomized trial evaluating ketamine for adult bronchoscopy. J Bronchology Interv Pulmonol. 2017;24(4):279–84.
20. Jose RJ, Shaefi S, Navani N. Anesthesia for bronchoscopy. Curr Opin Anaesthesiol. 2014;27(4):453–7.

21. Clark G, Licker M, Younossian AB, Soccal PM, Frey JG, Rochat T, et al. Titrated sedation with propofol or midazolam for flexible bronchoscopy: a randomised trial. Eur Respir J. 2009;34(6):1277–83.
22. Cai Y, Li W, Chen K. Efficacy and safety of spontaneous ventilation technique using dexmedetomidine for rigid bronchoscopic airway foreign body removal in children. Paediatr Anaesth. 2013;23(11):1048–53.
23. Pawlowski J. Anesthetic considerations for interventional pulmonary procedures. Curr Opin Anaesthesiol. 2013;26(1):6–12.
24. Sarkiss M, Kennedy M, Riedel B, Norman P, Morice R, Jimenez C, et al. Anesthesia technique for endobronchial ultrasound-guided fine needle aspiration of mediastinal lymph node. J Cardiothorac Vasc Anesth. 2007;21(6):892–6.
25. Ghorayeb BY, Shikhani AH. The use of dexamethasone in pediatric bronchoscopy. J Laryngol Otol. 1985;99(11):1127–9.
26. Wain JC Jr. Postintubation tracheal stenosis. Semin Thorac Cardiovasc Surg. 2009;21(3):284–9.
27. Espinoza A, Neumann K, Halvorsen PS, Sundset A, Kongerud J, Fosse E. Critical airway obstruction: challenges in airway management and ventilation during therapeutic bronchoscopy. J Bronchology Interv Pulmonol. 2015;22(1):41–7.
28. Pathak V, Welsby I, Mahmood K, Wahidi M, MacIntyre N, Shofer S. Ventilation and anesthetic approaches for rigid bronchoscopy. Ann Am Thorac Soc. 2014;11(4):628–34.
29. Murgu SD, Colt HG. Interventional bronchoscopy from bench to bedside: new techniques for central and peripheral airway obstruction. Clin Chest Med. 2010;31(1):101–15. Table of Contents
30. Erdos G, Tzanova I. Perioperative anaesthetic management of mediastinal mass in adults. Eur J Anaesthesiol. 2009;26(8):627–32.
31. Carter BW, Marom EM, Detterbeck FC. Approaching the patient with an anterior mediastinal mass: a guide for clinicians. J Thorac Oncol. 2014;9(9 Suppl 2):S102–9.
32. Azizad S, Sannananja B, Restrepo CS. Solid tumors of the mediastinum in adults. Semin Ultrasound CT MR. 2016;37(3):196–211.
33. Juan IC, Poorsattar SP, Banks DA, O'Brien EO, Fernando RJ, Addis D, et al. The anterior mediastinal mass-the challenging management of hypoxemia despite peripheral cannulation for ECMO. J Cardiothorac Vasc Anesth. 2021;35(10):3108–17.
34. Davis RD Jr, Oldham HN Jr, Sabiston DC Jr. Primary cysts and neoplasms of the mediastinum: recent changes in clinical presentation, methods of diagnosis, management, and results. Ann Thorac Surg. 1987;44(3):229–37.
35. Rubush JL, Gardner IR, Boyd WC, Ehrenhaft JL. Mediastinal tumors. Review of 186 cases. J Thorac Cardiovasc Surg. 1973;65(2):216–22.
36. Dubashi B, Cyriac S, Tenali SG. Clinicopathological analysis and outcome of primary mediastinal malignancies - a report of 91 cases from a single institute. Ann Thorac Med. 2009;4(3):140–2.
37. Azizkhan RG, Dudgeon DL, Buck JR, Colombani PM, Yaster M, Nichols D, et al. Life-threatening airway obstruction as a complication to the management of mediastinal masses in children. J Pediatr Surg. 1985;20(6):816–22.
38. Bechard P, Letourneau L, Lacasse Y, Cote D, Bussieres JS. Perioperative cardiorespiratory complications in adults with mediastinal mass: incidence and risk factors. Anesthesiology. 2004;100(4):826–34; discussion 5A
39. Anghelescu DL, Burgoyne LL, Liu T, Li CS, Pui CH, Hudson MM, et al. Clinical and diagnostic imaging findings predict anesthetic complications in children presenting with malignant mediastinal masses. Paediatr Anaesth. 2007;17(11):1090–8.
40. Dvorak P, Hoffmann P, Kocova E, Habal P, Nova M. CT-guided biopsy of the mediastinal masses. Can anatomical relationships predict complications? Biomed Pap Med Fac Univ Palacky Olomouc Czech Repub. 2019;163(3):220–6.
41. Garnon J, Ramamurthy N, Caudrelier JJ, Erceg G, Breton E, Tsoumakidou G, et al. MRI-guided percutaneous biopsy of mediastinal masses using a large bore magnet: technical feasibility. Cardiovasc Intervent Radiol. 2016;39(5):761–7.

42. Andersson T, Lindgren PG, Elvin A. Ultrasound guided tumour biopsy in the anterior mediastinum. An alternative to thoracotomy and mediastinoscopy. Acta Radiol. 1992;33(5):423–6.
43. Pullerits J, Holzman R. Anaesthesia for patients with mediastinal masses. Can J Anaesth. 1989;36(6):681–8.
44. Slinger P, Karsli C. Management of the patient with a large anterior mediastinal mass: recurring myths. Curr Opin Anaesthesiol. 2007;20(1):1–3.
45. Takeda S, Miyoshi S, Omori K, Okumura M, Matsuda H. Surgical rescue for life-threatening hypoxemia caused by a mediastinal tumor. Ann Thorac Surg. 1999;68(6):2324–6.
46. Anderson DM, Dimitrova GT, Awad H. Patient with posterior mediastinal mass requiring urgent cardiopulmonary bypass. Anesthesiology. 2011;114(6):1488–93.
47. Tempe DK, Arya R, Dubey S, Khanna S, Tomar AS, Grover V, et al. Mediastinal mass resection: femorofemoral cardiopulmonary bypass before induction of anesthesia in the management of airway obstruction. J Cardiothorac Vasc Anesth. 2001;15(2):233–6.
48. Dubey PK, Tripathi N. Anesthetic considerations in a patient with large anterior mediastinal mass. J Cardiothorac Vasc Anesth. 2019;33(4):1073–5.
49. Inoue M, Minami M, Shiono H, Miyoshi S, Takeda S, Ohta M, et al. Efficient clinical application of percutaneous cardiopulmonary support for perioperative management of a huge anterior mediastinal tumor. J Thorac Cardiovasc Surg. 2006;131(3):755–6.
50. Radvansky B, Hunt ML, Augoustides JG, Shah RM, Valentine EA, Kucharczuk JC, et al. Perioperative approaches to the anterior mediastinal mass-principles and pearls from a ten-year experience at an experienced referral center. J Cardiothorac Vasc Anesth. 2021;35(8):2503–12.
51. Hartigan PM, Ng JM, Gill RR. Anesthesia in a patient with a large mediastinal mass. N Engl J Med. 2018;379(6):587–8.
52. Hartigan PM, Karamnov S, Gill RR, Ng JM, Yacoubian S, Tsukada H, et al. Mediastinal masses, anesthetic interventions, and airway compression in adults: a prospective observational study. Anesthesiology. 2022;136(1):104–14.
53. Fiorelli A, Fiorito R, Messina G, Leone F, Mirra R, Pace MC, et al. Noninvasive positive pressure ventilation in the assessment of extrinsic tracheal stenosis. Interact Cardiovasc Thorac Surg. 2022;35(1)
54. Sarkiss M, Jimenez CA. The evolution of anesthesia management of patients with anterior mediastinal mass. Media. 2023;7:16.
55. Diaz Milian R, Foley E, Bauer M, Martinez-Velez A, Castresana MR. Expiratory central airway collapse in adults: anesthetic implications (part 1). J Cardiothorac Vasc Anesth. 2019;33(9):2546–54.
56. Boiselle PM, O'Donnell CR, Bankier AA, Ernst A, Millet ME, Potemkin A, et al. Tracheal collapsibility in healthy volunteers during forced expiration: assessment with multidetector CT. Radiology. 2009;252(1):255–62.
57. Ellingsen I, Holmedahl NH. Does excessive dynamic airway collapse have any impact on dynamic pulmonary function tests? J Bronchology Interv Pulmonol. 2014;21(1):40–6.
58. Boiselle PM, Litmanovich DE, Michaud G, Roberts DH, Loring SH, Womble HM, et al. Dynamic expiratory tracheal collapse in morbidly obese COPD patients. COPD. 2013;10(5):604–10.
59. Dal Negro RW, Tognella S, Guerriero M, Micheletto C. Prevalence of tracheobronchomalacia and excessive dynamic airway collapse in bronchial asthma of different severity. Multidiscip Respir Med. 2013;8(1):32.
60. Carden KA, Boiselle PM, Waltz DA, Ernst A. Tracheomalacia and tracheobronchomalacia in children and adults: an in-depth review. Chest. 2005;127(3):984–1005.
61. Morris MJ, Woods JT, McLaughlin CW. Exertional dyspnea and excessive dynamic airway collapse. Immunol Allergy Clin N Am. 2018;38(2):325–32.
62. Lee KS, Sun MRM, Ernst A, Feller-Kopman D, Majid A, Boiselle PM. Comparison of dynamic expiratory CT with bronchoscopy for diagnosing airway Malacia: a pilot evaluation. Chest. 2007;131(3):758–64.

63. Majid A, Gaurav K, Sanchez JM, Berger RL, Folch E, Fernandez-Bussy S, et al. Evaluation of tracheobronchomalacia by dynamic flexible bronchoscopy. A pilot study. Ann Am Thorac Soc. 2014;11(6):951–5.
64. Diaz Milian R, Foley E, Bauer M, Martinez-Velez A, Castresana MR. Expiratory central airway collapse in adults: corrective treatment (part 2). J Cardiothorac Vasc Anesth. 2019;33(9):2555–60.
65. Wright CD. Tracheobronchomalacia and expiratory collapse of central airways. Thorac Surg Clin. 2018;28(2):163–6.
66. Sonoda S, Sato K, Takagi Y, Sato Y, Murao F, Koide Y, et al. Undiagnosed tracheomalacia accompanied with accidental expiratory central airway collapse after tracheal intubation. Acute Med Surg. 2021;8(1):e665.
67. Bhagvandas J, Henry J. Tracheobronchomalacia causing end expiratory grunt post-intubation. Anaesth Rep. 2022;10(1):e12170.
68. Katoh H, Saitoh S, Takiguchi M, Yamasaki Y, Yamamoto M. A case of tracheomalacia during isoflurane anesthesia. Anesth Analg. 1995;80(5):1051–3.
69. Murakami S, Tsuruta S, Ishida K, Yamashita A, Matsumoto M. Excessive dynamic airway collapse during general anesthesia: a case report. JA Clin Rep. 2020;6(1):73.
70. Gaggini G, Nkamicaniye LM, Meyer S, Dubois PE. Expiratory central airway collapse during positive pressure ventilation: a case report. BMC Anesthesiol. 2022;22(1):50.
71. Lyaker MR, Davila VR, Papadimos TJ. Excessive dynamic airway collapse: an unexpected contributor to respiratory failure in a surgical patient. Case Rep Anesthesiol. 2015;2015:596857.
72. Zhu JH, Lei M, Chen EG, Qiao Q, Zhong TD. Ventilation strategy and anesthesia management in patients with severe tracheal stenosis undergoing urgent tracheal stenting. Acta Anaesthesiol Scand. 2018;62(5):600–7.
73. Markovitz BP, Randolph AG. Corticosteroids for the prevention and treatment of post-extubation stridor in neonates, children and adults. Cochrane Database Syst Rev. 2000;2:CD001000.
74. Doyle DJ, Hantzakos AG. Anesthetic management of the narrowed airway. Otolaryngol Clin N Am. 2019;52(6):1127–39.

Anesthesia for Patients with Anterior Mediastinal Mass Undergoing Interventional Pulmonary Procedures

8

Mona Sarkiss

8.1 Introduction

Mediastinal Anatomy The mediastinum is the central compartment of the chest cavity. Its boundaries are the sternum anteriorly, the spine posteriorly, the thoracic inlet superiorly, the diaphragm inferiorly, and the lung laterally. Theoretically, the mediastinum is divided by imaginary lines into superior and inferior compartments. The inferior compartment is further divided into anterior, posterior, and middle compartments [1]. The boundaries of the superior mediastinum are the thoracic inlet above and the sternal angle below, which is at the T4/T5 level posteriorly. The superior mediastinum contains vital organs such as the trachea, esophagus and thymus gland, great vessels aortic arch and its branches, the superior vena cava, brachiocephalic vein and the azygos vein and the vagus, phrenic, recurrent laryngeal nerve, the sympathetic trunk, and the cardiac plexus. The anterior mediastinal is encased between the sternum anteriorly and the pericardium posteriorly and contains the thymic remnants, fat, lymph nodes, and internal thoracic vessels. The middle mediastinum contains the heart, great vessels (ascending aorta, superior vena cave, and pulmonary artery and veins), the carina and the left and right main stem bronchi, the phrenic nerve, cardiac plexus, and lymph nodes. The posterior mediastinum is the space between the pericardium and the spine. The posterior mediastinum contains the esophagus, descending thoracic aorta, the azygos and hemiazygos veins, thoracic duct, the vagus and splanchnic nerves, as well as the sympathetic chain in addition to lymph nodes (Fig. 8.1).

Supplementary Information The online version contains supplementary material available at https://doi.org/10.1007/978-3-032-12007-6_8.

M. Sarkiss (✉)
Department of Anesthesiology and Perioperative Medicine, Department of Pulmonary Medicine, The University of Texas MD Anderson Cancer Center, Houston, TX, USA
e-mail: msarkiss@mdanderson.org

M. Sarkiss (ed.), *Anesthesia for Interventional Pulmonary Procedures*,
https://doi.org/10.1007/978-3-032-12007-6_8

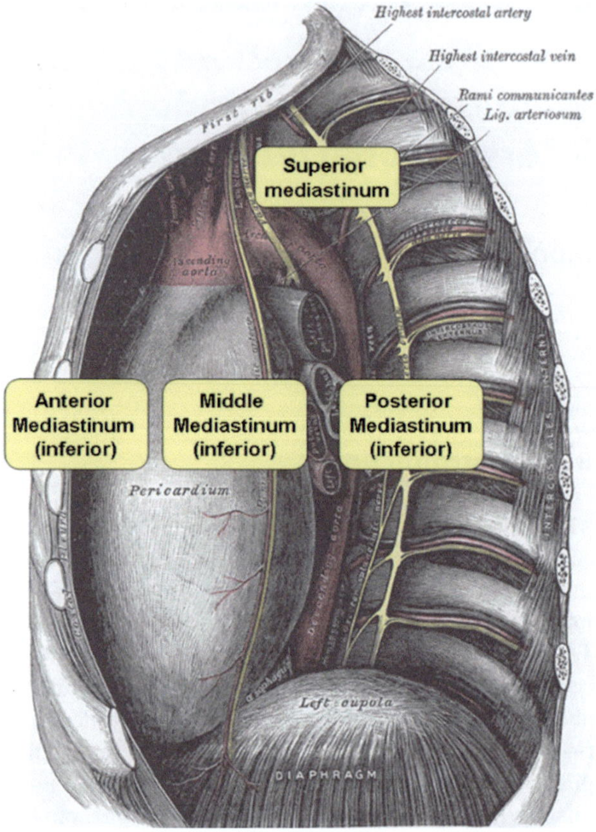

Fig. 8.1 Mediastinal anatomy. Annotated version of Gray's image 969; opened mediastinum viewed from the left body side

Benign and malignant growth within the compacted mediastinal spaces causes compression and compromise of its vital structures. The central airway, comprising the trachea, left and right mainstem bronchi, and their first bifurcation, can be compressed and compromised by pathological masses originating in the mediastinum. Common examples of such benign or malignant growth are thymomas, lymphomas, germ cell tumors, retrosternal thyroid parathyroid tumors in the superior and anterior mediastinum, and esophageal tumors, and neurologic tumors such as neurofibromas, schwannomas, and paragangliomas, as well as spinal tumors posteriorly.

8.2 Historical Perspective

Between the late 1960s and early 1970s, patients with Hodgkin's lymphomas were required to undergo staging laparotomy and splenectomy to define the extent of their disease and prescribe their treatment plan. A small number of these patients had mediastinal lymphoma growth with variable degrees of compression of the central airway and mediastinal vital structure. When routine anesthesia induction and endotracheal intubation techniques were used for the staging procedures, difficulties with ventilation and intubation were encountered. Case reports and small case series were published describing both successful and failed management of these patients, and some even reported death [2]. A review article published by Gordon in the International Anesthesiology Clinics Journal in 1972 was one of the earliest documentations of central airway obstruction due to compression by a mediastinal mass [3]. Dr. Gordon described several clinical assessment parameters that help evaluate the degree of airway obstruction in patients with mediastinal masses compressing the airway. He also offered several recommendations on how to safely manage these patients' airway during induction and maintenance of anesthesia.

In the following years, several recommendations for safe anesthesia induction and airway management continued to evolve and spread in the anesthesia community. These recommendations were based on case reports or small case series. The largest case series was published in 1976 where a retrospective review of 139 patients who underwent 203 surgical procedures for lymphoma staging was analyzed. Mediastinal mass was found in 74 patients, and preoperative evidence of airway obstruction was found in only 19 patients. Difficulties in intubation were encountered in 2 of the 19 patients with airway compression. This highlights the rarity of encountering patients with severe airway compromise by large mediastinal mass. Interestingly, both cases were managed successfully when the endotracheal tube was passed beyond the location of the airway narrowing. No catastrophic outcomes were reported in this case series [2].

Gordon's review article was likely the first to document the hypothesis that "In some cases, the induction of anesthesia and particularly the paralysis of the action of the voluntary muscles may result in collapse of the trachea and complete occlusion of the airway" [3]. This hypothesis was further emphasized by Bittar et al. in a case report where difficulty in ventilation was encountered after the patient with central airway compression was induced with morphine and thiopental, causing apnea and subsequent difficulty with assisted ventilation. An attempt to improve the ventilation by administration of succinylcholine infusion was futile. Bittar hypothesized that the paralysis of the smooth muscles in the airway caused airway collapse and further narrowing, making ventilation difficult, even though the difficulty in ventilation was initially encountered before the succinylcholine was administered [4]. These hypotheses resulted in the current recommendations and anesthesia practice techniques for induction and intubation of patients with mediastinal mass and airway compression. These recommendations included maintenance of spontaneous ventilation, avoidance of muscle relaxation during induction of general anesthesia, and the preferred utilization of inhalation induction of general anesthesia. Further recommendations to manage the airway if ventilation difficulties are encountered included changing the patient position to relieve the airway compression, discontinuation of general anesthesia and waking the patient from general anesthesia, or performing the procedures under local anesthesia. Other recommendations were to delay the procedure until the patient receives radiotherapy and the size of the mediastinal mass and degree of airway compression are reduced [5]. It is important to note that an interventional pulmonary procedure to reestablish the airway patency can be a lifesaving safe bridge to undergo medical and radiation therapy in patients with severe respiratory distress and delaying the procedure might not be optimal in such circumstances.

Gordon's and Bittar's hypotheses and their resultant recommendations remained and were reiterated in multiple publications since. Only recently these hypotheses were challenged, and doubt was shed on their accompanying recommendations in an elegant study by Hartigan in *Anesthesiology* and *New England Journal of Medicine* [6, 7]. Initially, Hartigan published a case report in 2018 where a patient with anterior mediastinal mass compressing the airway was intubated awake in a semi-sitting position and a video bronchoscopy was inserted at the level of the carina before general anesthesia was induced and muscle relaxation was administered. Hartigan noted that there was an increase of the airway caliber after the institution of positive pressure ventilation and further improvement after the addition of muscle paralysis [7]. Hartigan followed this case report with a small single-center prospective observations study to document the changes in the caliber of the central airway in 17 patients with mediastinal mass and central airway compression in 2022. Of the 17 patients, 12 were diagnosed with anterior mediastinal mass, 1 posterior mass, and 3 with both anterior and posterior mediastinal mass. All patients were intubated with 8.5 ETT or LMA awake after topicalization of the upper airway with local anesthesia. Using video bronchoscopy, the authors observed and measured changes in the caliber of the obstructed airway in awake spontaneously ventilating patients, anesthetized spontaneously ventilating patients and anesthetized patients with positive pressure ventilation before and after muscle relaxation was administered. The findings of this study were surprising as no changes in the narrowed airway caliber were noted between awake and anesthetized spontaneously ventilating patients. However, it was noted that the airway caliber increased after the implementation of positive pressure ventilation and further improved after the addition of a muscle relaxant [6].

During the same year, a study by Fiorelli measuring peak inspiratory flow (PIF) and peak expiratory flow (PEF) in 13 patients with anterior mediastinal mass requiring tracheal stenting was published. The patients were supine, and a face mask connected to an anesthesia ventilator circuit was securely placed on their face. The PIF and PEF were recorded while the patients are spontaneously ventilating and after the addition of noninvasive positive pressure (NIPPV) ventilator with PEEP of 10. The study showed that central tracheal compression by mediastinal mas impaired the PIF more the PEF and increased the PEF:PIF ratio in awake spontaneously ventilating patients. An improvement in both the PIF and PEF was noted after the addition of NIPPV and PEEP 10 with improvement in the PEF:PIF ratio [8]. This publication complemented Hartigan's study by demonstrating that positive pressure ventilation improved both inspiratory and expiratory flows in awake patients with central airway compression by mediastinal mass [9].

These findings have significant implication that will be discussed further in the anesthesia management section of this chapter. It is noteworthy that to date no randomized controlled studies have been published to support or defy the current practices and recommendation for management of patients with mediastinal mass and airway compression.

8.3 Preoperative Assessment

8.3.1 Patient History

A detailed patient's history is essential to gauge the degree and severity of the compression of the central airway and other vital organs by the mediastinal mass. The patients' symptoms can range from dyspnea with exertion to dyspnea at rest. Gordon's review article was the earliest to report that in an otherwise healthy patient symptoms of respiratory distress at rest are encountered when the tracheal lumen is narrowed down to 3–4 mm. A clinical assessment tool that remains standing to this day is where airway narrowing beyond 5 mm is considered critical and is associated with severe respiratory distress at rest [10, 11]. Significant compression of the recurrent laryngeal nerves presents with hoarseness, difficulty speaking, and choking on food. Esophageal compression can present with difficulty in swallowing, ranging from dysphagia to solid and liquids to inability to swallow the saliva. Symptoms of cardiac and major vessels compression should be suspected when symptoms such as palpitations, facial swelling, and episodes of dizziness, especially with coughing or straining, are reported. Orthopnea or positional dyspnea in a patient with mediastinal mass can have multiple etiologies such as pericardial effusion or significant airway compression by the mass.

8.3.2 Physical Exam

Vital signs can reflect the degree of hypoxemia and hypercarbia in patients with central airway compression. For example, tachycardia, atrial flutter, atrial fibrillation, hyper- or hypotension, and low saturation are common signs. Basic signs of respiratory distress such as nasal ala flaring, and suprasternal and intercostal retraction should be sought. Compression of other vital structure such as the esophagus and the superior vena cava can be evident by dysphagia, inability to swallow the saliva, and facial and/or upper extremity swelling, respectively. Compression or tumor infiltration of the recurrent laryngeal nerve manifests as progressive hoarseness, inspiratory stridor, and vocal cord paralysis seen on nasopharyngeal bronchoscopic inspection. Chest auscultation can reveal both inspiratory and or expiratory wheezing, and loss of breath sounds distal to the obstructed airway in areas of collapsed lung or diminished breath sounds under pleural effusions.

8.3.3 Imaging

In his review, Gordon recommended the utilization of preoperative chest X-ray to assess the diameter of the trachea before the procedure. In our modern era, chest CT scan and 3-D reconstruction of the central airway can give accurate information about the degree of airway narrowing as well as the location and length of the segment of the airway affected. Knowing the degree of airway narrowing, location, and length of the narrowed segment is essential in planning the anesthesia induction technique, method of ventilation and airway device to be used at different stages of the procedure [10].

8.3.4 Laboratory

Baseline complete blood count (CBC) and chemistry, in addition to coagulation studies, can shed light on the patient's status, for example, anemia related to bleeding, or poor nutritional status, elevated white blood count WBCs related to postobstructive pneumonia, preprocedure transfusion, and correction of coagulopathy might be needed if tumor debulking is planned. Blood chemistry is also essential to identify and correct electrolyte imbalances related to paraneoplastic syndromes, for example, hyponatremia, hypokalemia, and hyperkalemia. Severe airway obstruction might also be associated with chronic carbon dioxide retention and elevated bicarbonate levels detected on arterial blood gas analysis as acute or chronic respiratory acidosis.

8.4 Interventional Pulmonary Procedures

Patients with central airway obstruction due to mediastinal mass compression are referred to the interventional pulmonologists for stent placement with or without tumor debulking to relieve the airway obstruction. Stenting the narrowed airway is vital as it acts as a bridge to enhance the patient's respiratory status while undergoing treatment for the mediastinal mass, for example, chemotherapy, immunotherapy, radiation therapy, and/or surgery. Occasionally, the stenting procedure is performed for a palliative indication to reduce the respiratory distress while the patient is transitioning to hospice care.

Rigid bronchoscopy is the most valuable tool for patients with central airway obstruction by mediastinal mass undergoing interventional pulmonary procedures. Once introduced in the airway, the rigid bronchoscope can be advanced distally to bypass the area of the obstruction and immediately reinstate a patent airway. Stenting the airway open with the rigid bronchoscope is lifesaving, especially if ventilation difficulties are encountered.

The procedure commonly begins with bronchoscopic airway exam to assess the location and extent of the airway narrowing and/or the presence of endoluminal tumor requiring debulking. Measurements are taken of the narrowed segment of the airway to select the appropriate type and size of the airway stent needed. Both silicone stents and self-expanding metal stents (SEM) can be used to expand the obstructed segment of the airway. Occasionally, Y-silicon stent is needed when a central obstruction involves the main carina. Balloon dilation of the self-expanding metal stents may be needed to further open the stent and improve the airway caliber. Occasionally, biopsy of the tumor invading and/or compressing the airway is performed to aid in the diagnosis of the lesion. Endobronchial biopsies are performed if there is tumor invasion of the airway and ultrasound-guided transbronchial biopsies for external tumor causing central airway compression may be needed. Endobronchial ultrasound-guided transbronchial needle aspiration of the mediastinal lymph can also be performed if mediastinal staging is indicated.

8.5 Anesthesia Management

8.5.1 Anesthesia Induction

Historically, bypassing the anesthesia induction and proceeding with awake intubation after airway topicalization or inhalation induction and maintenance of spontaneous ventilation has been the recommended practice [12]. These recommendations are not suited for interventional pulmonary procedures where insertion of the rigid bronchoscopy is needed. Awake intubation with the rigid bronchoscope is not practiced for obvious reasons. Similarly, inhalation induction cannot be used with rigid bronchoscopy due to the leak of the anesthesia gas from the open ports of the rigid bronchoscope, causing room air contamination and inconsistent delivery of the required MAC of the inhalation agents. This leaves us with total Intravenous anesthesia as the most suited anesthesia induction method for interventional pulmonary procedures where the rigid bronchoscope is used.

Preoxygenation is essential and recommended by the American Society of Anesthesiologists (ASA) in their difficult airway management algorithm [13]. Patients with central airway compression by mediastinal mass may not have a difficult upper airway per se but ventilation and intubation difficulties are anticipated, making the patient's lower/central airway difficult. Preoxygenation can be performed in the sitting or semi-sitting position where the patient has the best ability to breathe with the least discomfort.

Monitoring with the standard ASA monitors with consideration for additional monitors as bispectral index (BIS) and noninvasive and invasive arterial line monitoring can be used as indicated. BIS can help titrate the intravenous anesthetic to obtain the appropriate depth of anesthesia while minimizing hypotension.

Anesthesia induction in patients in respiratory distress is known to be associated with hypotension and has been coined as "the physiologically difficult airway," thus, necessitating slow induction titration while optimization the patient's volume status [14, 15]. Slow intravenous induction with propofol infusion while maintaining high fractional inspired oxygen (FiO2) and intravenous fluid for volume resuscitation can be used. Avoidance of additional induction agents known to induce hypotension should be considered, for example, narcotics.

8.5.2 Ventilation

Historical ventilatory recommendations for patients with mediastinal mass compressing the airway remain valuable today. These recommendations are:

Avoid hyperventilation Gordon recognized that the degree of tracheal airway obstruction is influenced by the respiratory rate, tidal volume, patient's position, and phase of respiration. He had specific recommendations to avoid hyperventilation once the patient is intubated. He documented his rationale to avoid hyperventilation by stating that "patients with chronic obstruction of the trachea may have compensated respiratory acidosis and high $PaCO_2$. Hyperventilation will cause an abrupt and significant reduction of the carbon dioxide, resulting in metabolic alkalosis, which in some instances will result in the reduction of the cardiac output, collapse of the cardiovascular homeostatic mechanisms and cardiac arrest" [3].

Prolonged expiratory phase An early case report of successful management of a young patient with mediastinal mass causing severe symptoms related to tracheal and bilateral main stem narrowing was published in the *British Journal of Anesthesia* in 1973. The patient was electively intubated with the tip of the ETT positioned in the right main stem distal to the obstruction. The patient was maintained on mechanical ventilation while he received four cycles of radiotherapy over a 4-day period. The patient was then successfully extubated as the tumor shrank post radiation. The author emphasized the importance of using a prolonged expiratory phase during the 4 days of mechanical ventilation. He stated his rationale as "to ensure complete expiration, however, an unusually long expiration time is necessary. In addition, marked hypotension may occur as a result of the high intrathoracic pressure, and the danger of progression to complete airway obstruction is always present." This was the first published recommendation to increase the I:E ratio in patients with airway compression by mediastinal mass to avoid air trapping and lung hyperinflation with subsequent difficulty in ventilation due to high airway pressure and hemodynamic collapse [16].

After anesthesia induction and the BIS monitor decreases to indicate deep sedation levels and the lash reflex is lost, the anesthesia mask can be secured on the patients face and ventilation is controlled. Volume-controlled ventilatory mode with I:E ratio of 1:4 can be used. As per Hartigan's study, the positive pressure can increase the narrowed airway diameter and allow for ventilation. A high I:E ratio, for example, 1:4, allows for prolonged exhalation and minimization of air trapping distal to the area of obstruction as described previously in the review article by Gordon. Low respiratory rates 8–10 breath/min further increase the expiratory time and prevent air trapping.

The adequacy of ventilation at this point can be determined by observing the expired tidal volume of the ventilator screen. Once an expired tidal volume reading is detected on the anesthesia machine monitor indicating the ability to ventilate past the airway obstruction, a muscle relaxant such as rocuronium or cisatracurium can be safely administered to facilitate the insertion of the rigid bronchoscope without causing injury to the vocal cord and trachea. Jet ventilation or mechanical/assisted ventilation can be used through the rigid bronchoscope [9]. Once the rigid bronchoscope is inserted past the area of obstruction, ventilation becomes easier and any trapped air is released.

8.5.3 Airway Devices

History Gordon advocated for ETT placement in patients with central airway obstruction. He recommended to select the appropriate size of the ETT based on the estimated degree of tracheal obstruction noted on a baseline chest X-ray. He went on to recommend the insertion of an ETT after topicalization of the airway with local anesthetics in a conscious spontaneously ventilating patient [3]. Gordon also described the importance of the insertion of the ETT past the area of narrowing in the trachea and advocated for the use of a bronchoscope to ensure that the tip of the ETT is appropriately positioned distal to the obstruction. He went on to recommend the use of bronchoscopic-guided intubation if difficulty is encountered in passing the ETT through the tracheal narrowing.

ETT is coined as the most secure airway device as it ensures adequate delivery of ventilation while protecting the airway from soiling in the event of aspiration. The utility of ETT during interventional pulmonary procedures has been challenged as the location of the ETT may obscure and/or cause trauma to the narrowed airway or tumors in the airway. This is especially true in tumors or tumor compression of the upper and middle third of the trachea. Additionally, the small caliber of the ETT compared to a rigid bronchoscope will limit the type and number of interventional pulmonary instruments needed to reestablish the airway patency making such critical procedure even more difficult. It is noteworthy that silicon stents can only be deployed via the rigid bronchoscope due to the rigid nature of its deployment device. Meanwhile, self-expanding metal stents can be deployed through and ETT or supraglottic airway device.

Supraglottic airway (SGA) The laryngeal mask airway (LMA) was first introduced in the United States in 1992. The LMA has gained great popularity among interventional pulmonologist as it allows for complete inspection of the airway from the vocal cord down to the distal airway as well as the free mobility of the bronchoscope, especially the larger diameter therapeutic bronchoscope, in the airway. Reports of using an SGA during airway exam and management of patients with mediastinal mass have been reported. However, a precautionary statement is that high airway pressure in patients with central airway narrowing may exceed the pressure at which air leak is encountered with the SGA [10]. It is noteworthy that a case report documented adequate ventilation through an SGA in a patient with 90% tracheal obstruction by a mediastinal mass [17].

The rigid bronchoscope maybe the safest airway device in patients with mediastinal mass causing central airway narrowing. As stated previously, the rigid bronchoscope has multiple advantages in the management, ventilation, and re-establishing airway patency in patients with central airway obstruction by mediastinal mass [18]. These advantages include

- Stenting the airway open by bypassing the narrow airway segment.
- Allow for a safe and adequate jet ventilation at the higher pressures needed to widen and traverse the narrowed airway without causing barotrauma. To avoid barotrauma during jet ventilation with high pressure, the proximal end of the rigid bronchoscope must remain open to air without the application of caps.
- Deployment of a silicon stent or a Y-stent can only be performed through the rigid bronchoscope.
- The rigid bronchoscope allows for the simultaneous insertion of multiple instruments if needed to recanalize the airway.
- The rigid bronchoscope can be used to tamponade bleeding areas by direct compression.

8.5.4 ECMO

Several published case reports describe the use of ECMO as the main source of oxygenation or a rescue method in patients with mediastinal mass undergoing surgery and interventional bronchoscopy procedures. One interesting case report describes a patient with >90% tracheal obstruction by mediastinal mass undergoing surgical tumor debulking and insertion of tracheal stent [17]. The SVC patency was confirmed radiologically before the internal jugular vein and left femoral veins were cannulated. Anesthesia was then induced, SGA was inserted, and a pressure-controlled ventilation ensued. The tumor was resected, and a tracheal stent was placed before the patient was awakened from general anesthesia. This case report is significant as it was the first to document the ability to obtain adequate positive pressure ventilation through SGA in a patient with > 90% tracheal stenosis. Additionally, this case emphasized the valuable role of ECMO in maintaining oxygenation and hemodynamics in patients undergoing surgery for severe central airway obstruction. Additional publications have recommended the use of ECMO in patients with central airway obstruction with cardiac involvement [19, 20].

8.5.5 Extubation and Recovery

At the end of the procedure where the airway patency has been established, transitioning from the rigid bronchoscope to SGA can be performed. Endotracheal intubation as a transition from rigid bronchoscopy is not recommended as the ETT can dislodge the tracheal stent or cause its collapse. Additionally, reports of inadvertently inserting the tip of the ETT between the tracheal wall and the stent causing difficulty in ventilation have been reported. Once the airway is established, discontinuation of the intravenous anesthetic and reversal of the muscle paralysis can ensue. The patient is extubated when extubation criteria are met as per routine anesthesia practice. Some centers transition from the rigid bronchoscope to a face mask after muscle relaxant reversal and return of spontaneous ventilation [21]. The patients can then be transitioned to the recovery room with supplemental oxygen.

In the recovery room, the patients are monitored with standard monitoring while the supplemental oxygen is weaned down as per common practice. It is important to note that airway procedures are not associated with pain and narcotics may not be necessary, especially in this population of patients with airway compromise. However, sore throat related to the rigid bronchoscope insertion and airway management might be encountered. Once adequate recovery criteria are met, the patient can be discharged.

Immediate and delayed postprocedure complications related to the procedure and general anesthesia can be encountered. These complications are rare but worth mentioning due to the grave effect they have on the patient [22]. Examples are

- Respiratory failure secondary to.
  - Stent migration.
  - Stent obstruction by thick secretions, blood clots, or residual tumor growth.
  - Narcotic administration and residual general anesthetics.
- Airway perforation during stent placement or by pressure necrosis exerted by the stent. This may present as pneumomediastinum, surgical emphysema, pneumothorax, or delayed mediastinitis.
- Upper airway and tongue injuries during rigid bronchoscope insertion.

8.5.6 Mediastinal Mass with Cardiac Involvement

Death in a patient with mediastinal mass at the time of anesthesia induction was reported in a 9-year-old boy in 1981 [23]. It was intriguing that no difficulty in ventilation was encountered at the time of induction. However, post-induction the patient became cyanotic and suffered bradycardia followed by cardiac arrest and unsuccessful CPR. The patients' baseline history indicated cyanosis and syncope while the child is bearing down with bowel movement. Postmortem exam showed a large mediastinal mass encasing the heart and infiltrating the pericardium. This case report highlights the importance of preoperative assessment of cardiac and great vessels involvement in patients with mediastinal mass. Symptoms of syncope while bearing down herald the detrimental effects of increased intrathoracic pressure with bearing down on the compressed heart and major vessels. It should also alert the anesthesiologist that positive pressure ventilation might have a similar detrimental effect on the circulation under general anesthesia with positive pressure ventilation. These cases are best managed with ECMO support as described above.

8.5.7 Posterior Mediastinal Mass

The observation of increase in airway caliber with institution of positive pressure ventilation can be partially explained by the pliability of the posterior tracheal membrane. The wall of the trachea is made of C-shaped incomplete cartilaginous rings anteriorly and laterally and a posterior membrane making the trachea a semi-rigid

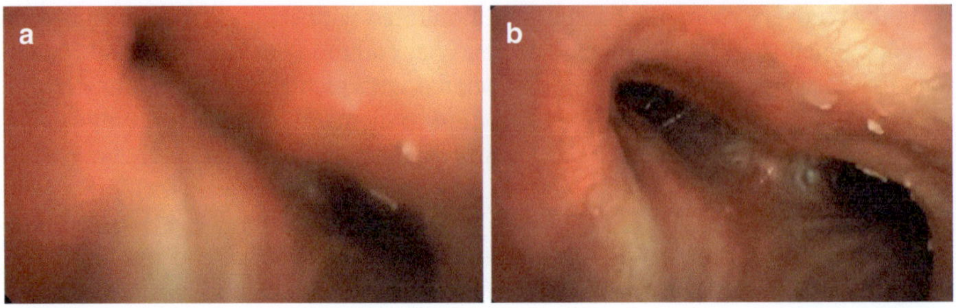

Fig. 8.2 Increase in the airway caliber with positive pressure ventilation: (**a**) during expiration; (**b**) during jet ventilation

structure. The posterior tracheal membrane is made of smooth muscle (Trachealis) lined with mucous membrane and ciliated epithelium. Contraction of the posterior membrane muscle constricts the tracheal lumen to build up pressure to generate forceful expiration to aid with coughing and clearance of secretion. Alternatively, positive pressure ventilation can cause posterior displacement of the posterior tracheal membrane, leading to increase in the caliber of the tracheal lumen. This observation is the basis for using noninvasive positive pressure ventilation such as CPAP in patients with dynamic airway collapse as the positive pressure stents the tracheal lumen open. In patients with anterior mediastinal mass, an increase in the compressed tracheal lumen caliber with positive pressure ventilation may be contributed to posterior displacement of the posterior tracheal membrane (Fig. 8.2 and Video 8.1). Patients with posterior mediastinal mass compressing and limiting the expansion of the posterior tracheal membrane might cause increased ventilation difficulties with positive pressure ventilation compared to patients with anterior mediastinal mass with freely mobile posterior membrane.

8.6 Summary

Mediastinal mass causing central airway compression has been a challenge to the induction of anesthesia and intubation. Multiple case reports and case series have warned of the detrimental outcomes of general anesthesia in this patient's population. Recent investigations have shed light on the mechanics of airway and airflow in a patient with central airway obstruction with mediastinal mass. Understanding the effect of positive pressure ventilation and muscle paralysis on the airway caliber led to new safe anesthesia induction and ventilation recommendations in patients with central airway obstruction. Future prospective randomized trials are needed to further examine and refine these new recommendations.

References

1. Stoddard N, Heil JR, Lowery DR. Anatomy, thorax, Mediastinum. In: StatPearls. Treasure Island (FL); 2025.
2. Piro AJ, Weiss DR, Hellman S. Mediastinal Hodgkin's disease: a possible danger for intubation anesthesia. Intubation danger in Hodgkin's disease. Int J Radiat Oncol Biol Phys. 1976;1(5–6):415–9.
3. Gordon RA. Anesthetic management of patients with airway problems. Int Anesthesiol Clin. 1972;10(3):37–59.
4. Bittar D. Respiratory obstruction associated with induction of general anesthesia in a patient with mediastinal Hodgkin's disease. Anesth Analg. 1975;54(3):399–403.
5. Blank RS, de Souza DG. Anesthetic management of patients with an anterior mediastinal mass: continuing professional development. Can J Anaesth. 2011;58(9):853–9. 60–7
6. Hartigan PM, Karamnov S, Gill RR, Ng JM, Yacoubian S, Tsukada H, et al. Mediastinal masses, anesthetic interventions, and airway compression in adults: a prospective observational study. Anesthesiology. 2022;136(1):104–14.
7. Hartigan PM, Ng JM, Gill RR. Anesthesia in a patient with a large mediastinal mass. N Engl J Med. 2018;379(6):587–8.
8. Fiorelli A, Fiorito R, Messina G, Leone F, Mirra R, Pace MC, et al. Noninvasive positive pressure ventilation in the assessment of extrinsic tracheal stenosis. Interact Cardiovasc Thorac Surg. 2022;35(1)
9. Sarkiss M, Jimenez CA. The evolution of anesthesia management of patients with anterior mediastinal mass. Mediastinum. 2023;7:16.
10. Espinoza A, Neumann K, Halvorsen PS, Sundset A, Kongerud J, Fosse E. Critical airway obstruction: challenges in airway management and ventilation during therapeutic bronchoscopy. J Bronchol Interv Pulmonol. 2015;22(1):41–7.
11. Conacher ID. Anaesthesia and tracheobronchial stenting for central airway obstruction in adults. Br J Anaesth. 2003;90(3):367–74.
12. Hachenberg T, Schilling T, Kretzschmar M. Perioperative management of patients with mediastinal mass syndrome. Curr Opin Anaesthesiol. 2025;38(1):58–64.
13. Apfelbaum JL, Hagberg CA, Connis RT, Abdelmalak BB, Agarkar M, Dutton RP, et al. 2022 American Society of Anesthesiologists Practice Guidelines for Management of the Difficult Airway. Anesthesiology. 2022;136(1):31–81.
14. Mosier JM, Joshi R, Hypes C, Pacheco G, Valenzuela T, Sakles JC. The physiologically difficult airway. West J Emerg Med. 2015;16(7):1109–17.
15. Mosier JM. Physiologically difficult airway in critically ill patients: winning the race between haemoglobin desaturation and tracheal intubation. Br J Anaesth. 2020;125(1):e1–4.
16. Amaha K, Okutsu Y, Nakamura Y. Major airway obstruction by mediastinal tumour. A case report. Br J Anaesth. 1973;45(10):1082–4.
17. Landa AB, Krishnamurthy K, Goldman HS. A right para-tracheal mass extending into the anterior mediastinum: an anesthetic management conundrum. Ann Card Anaesth. 2021;24(3):381–3.
18. Sarkiss M, Eapen GA. Airway management for central airway and transbronchial lung procedures. Curr Anesthesiol Rep. 2022;12(3):390–7.
19. Meyer S, Dincq AS, Pirard L, Ocak S, D'Odemont JP, Eucher P, et al. Bronchotracheal stenting management by rigid bronchoscopy under extracorporeal membrane oxygenation (ECMO) support: 10 years of experience in a tertiary center. Can Respir J. 2021;2021:8822591.
20. Nokes BT, Vaszar L, Jahanyar J, Swanson KL. VV-ECMO-assisted high-risk endobronchial stenting as rescue for asphyxiating mediastinal mass. J Bronchol Interv Pulmonol. 2018;25(2):144–7.

21. Matus I, Wilton S, Ho E, Raja H, Feng L, Murgu S, et al. Current practices supporting rigid bronchoscopy-an international survey. J Bronchol Interv Pulmonol. 2023;30(4):328–34.
22. Ost DE, Ernst A, Grosu HB, Lei X, Diaz-Mendoza J, Slade M, et al. Complications following therapeutic bronchoscopy for malignant central airway obstruction: results of the AQuIRE registry. Chest. 2015;148(2):450–71.
23. Keon TP. Death on induction of anesthesia for cervical node biopsy. Anesthesiology. 1981;55(4):471–2.

Anesthesia for Interventional Pulmonary Management of Patients with Airway Fistulas

9

Prarthna Chandar, Basvana Goudra, and Divakara Gouda

9.1 Introduction

An abnormal connection between two structures or organs or between an organ and body surface is referred to as fistula [1]. Airway fistulas are generally connections between bronchus or trachea and the surrounding structures with potential or true space. These include pleural space (bronchopleural fistula) or esophagus (tracheoesophageal fistula, bronchoesophageal fistula) or stomach (gastrobronchial fistula, gastrotracheal fistula). Cancer (typically esophageal), trauma, and prolonged endotracheal intubation are a few of the common causes. The consequences of such fistula depend on the location, cause, and the resulting changes in the anatomy and physiology of the adjoining structures. Recurrent pulmonary infections and sepsis are possible. Other undesirable effects are poor oxygenation, ineffective ventilation, and airway obstruction. Other types such as parenchymal and aortic fistulas airways are very rare and often fatal. Significant advances in understanding the pathophysiology and technological advances have allowed pulmonologists to create a management plan that allow better quality of life. The anesthesia challenges depend on the nature of fistulous connection and the associated morbidity.

P. Chandar (✉)
Department of Pulmonology, Sidney Kimmel Medical College, Philadelphia, PA, USA
e-mail: Prarthna.Chandar@jefferson.edu

B. Goudra
Department of Anesthesiology, Sidney Kimmel Medical College, Jefferson Health, Philadelphia, PA, USA

D. Gouda
PGY1, Internal Medicine, Inspira Health Network, Mullica Hill, NJ, USA

M. Sarkiss (ed.), *Anesthesia for Interventional Pulmonary Procedures*,
https://doi.org/10.1007/978-3-032-12007-6_9

9.2 Communications Between Bronchus and Pleural Space

An abnormal communication between the bronchial tree and the pleural space is referred to as a bronchopleural fistula (BPF). If the communication is visible during bronchoscopy, it is referred to as central BPF, while if it is not visible on bronchoscopy, it is called a peripheral BPF. Further, a communication between the lung parenchyma distal to the segmental bronchus and the pleural space is called alveolar pleural fistula (APF) [2].

9.2.1 Causes of Bronchopleural Fistula

Prolonged postoperative air leak (an air leak lasting beyond postoperative day 5) with BPF frequently occurs after lung resection surgery [3]. In fact, the most frequent postoperative complication after elective lung resection is an alveolar-pleural fistula [4, 5]. Although around 50% of patients develop air leak after lung resections, they rarely require specific treatment and typically resolve in a couple of days [5]. Presence of a low predicted postoperative forced expiratory volume in 1 s and upper lobe surgery increases the risk of BPF. In a retrospective study of Sirbu et al., 4.4% (22/490) of the patients undergoing lung resection for non-small cell lung carcinoma developed BPF. They documented that comorbidities such as diabetes, frailty, and steroid treatment increased the risk of fistula development [6]. BPF was also observed more frequently after right-sided pneumonectomy, especially if postoperative ventilation was required. Higher preoperative radiation exposure is a risk factor for BPF after right pneumonectomy, whereas carinal closure exerts a protective effect [7]. In another study involving 221 pneumonectomies for non-small cell lung carcinoma, multivariate analysis showed that preoperative respiratory infection and right pneumonectomy were the only independent risk factors for BPF development [8]. Although the incidence of BPF after pneumonectomy could be as high as 20%, neoadjuvant immunotherapy is likely to reduce these rates as the need for such extensive surgery will recede [9, 10]. A vast majority of the leaks occur at the stump closure site, likely to be related to infection, ischemic necrosis, and poor secretion clearance [11].

Necrotizing pneumonias are another group that can cause BPF [12–16]. Many bacteria, viruses, and fungi are implicated. These include both aerobic and anerobic organisms, including rare forms such as *Mycobacterium avium* complex. Both blunt and penetrating lung injuries are another group of causes. Rarely BPF can follow procedures such as lung biopsy, chest tube drainage, thoracocentesis, chemical pneumonitis (such as kerosine), or radiation therapy [17].

In a retrospective study involving 4794 consecutive patients who underwent lung resections, Matsunaga et al. observed BPF in 32 patients (0.67%) [18]. Male sex, obesity, low vital capacity, type of resection (right lower lobectomy, right middle and lower lobectomy at lower risk than right pneumonectomy), and additional resection of surrounding organs were major risk factors. 15.6% die within 90 days and about 28% in 5 years. In another 10 years (September 2012–August 2021), in an institution-based multicenter retrospective cohort study [19] from Ethiopia, of the 2546 patients admitted to the cardiothoracic unit in three hospitals, 52(2%) developed/had BPF, of which two-thirds were male. While 31 (60%) were spontaneous, the remainder were postsurgical, 1 being post-traumatic.

Peripheral bronchopleural fistulas are typically caused by surgery, bronchiectasis, necrotizing pneumonia and abscess, cancer, tuberculosis, infarction, penetrating trauma, and barotrauma [20].

9.2.2 Anatomy, Mechanism, and Clinical Presentation

As mentioned earlier, BPF is a fistulous communication between the bronchus and the pleural space. The breached portion of the lung tissue (bronchus of any segment, depending on the cause) opens into the pleural space, where the pressure is normally negative (−3 to −5 cm H2O). BPF indicates a breakdown of the bronchial stump. If the bronchus is already inflamed (as in tuberculosis), poor nutritional status, or cancer, chances of breakdown are higher [21]. Reinforcing the bronchial stump reduces the risk.

Most commonly, diagnosis of a fistula is made between 10 and 15 days (can develop up to 3 months after a lung resection). It is usually related to breach in the suture or staple line. A proposed classification of these fistula based on the time of onset is as follows: early: 1–7 days after surgery; intermediate: 8–30 days after surgery; and late: more than 30 days after surgery [22]. Productive cough, shortness of breath, fever, pus draining from the chest wall (empyema), and respiratory distress are some of the clinical presentations in that order of frequency [19]. In a chart review of 17 BPF patients (2 were post-pneumonectomy and 15 were post-lobectomy), Boudaya observed that the mean interval between surgery and fistula development was 20 days (range, 5–270 days) [23].

A chest X-ray is often the first investigation ordered, and the findings depend on the cause. In patients who had pneumonectomy (a common cause), an acute decrease in the pleural fluid level or disappearance of pleural fluid is seen [19]. In those with a subacute presentation (productive cough, fever, leukocytosis), a new air-fluid level appears in a previously opacified hemothorax. In a series of 17 patients, Boudaya et al. observed hydropneumothorax ($n = 6$), empyema ($n = 8$), atelectasis ($n = 1$), and persistent pleural detachment on chest X-ray [23]. A CT scan may also reveal pneumothorax, pneumomediastinum, and underlying lung pathology. In addition, an actual fistulous communication could be seen as well. Actual localization of the fistula (and diagnosis confirmation) requires fiberoptic bronchoscopy [19]. In one case series of 17 patients, the median diameter of the BPF orifice was 3.3 mm (range, 2–9 mm). Of these, 15 patients had a fistula of 5 mm or smaller and the same number had on the right side [23].

Persistent air leak and a prolonged pneumothorax combined with a pleural effusion (hydropneumothorax) are some of the clinical presentations of peripheral bronchopleural fistulas. Aspiration pneumonia is possible and is caused by the pus flowing backward through the bronchus from an empyema [20]. An apparent continuation of a bronchus or the lung parenchyma to the pleural space on a CT scan provides definite evidence of a peripheral BPF. These findings are present in about 50%. Any hydropneumothorax should encourage a CT evaluation to search for peripheral BPF [20].

9.2.3 Nonsurgical Interventional Management

A conservative approach may be appropriate at the beginning and includes drainage of the infected pleural space, prophylactic antibiotics, and adequate clearance of bronchial secretions [23]. If the fistula does not close spontaneously, the options are attempts to close the fistula with bronchoscopy or by surgical means. Depending on the patient's physical status, location, and size of the fistula, many bronchoscopic interventions are available.

In a retrospective chart review of patients who developed post-lobectomy bronchopleural fistula, Spanish investigators concluded that conservative treatment of post-lobectomy bronchopleural fistula is a safe and simple option that must be borne in mind and applied as necessary [24]. Of the seven cases of fistula developed after 1373 lobectomies (6 mm to suture dehiscence, diagnosed by endoscopic visualization), six underwent conservative treatment that consisted of insertion of a thoracostomy drainage tube in the pleural cavity, with either no aspiration or with the minimum aspiration necessary to get the lung expanded, while one initially underwent bronchoscopic stent placement to facilitate mechanical ventilation, with no success. Whenever possible, thoracostomy tube was connected to a Heimlich valve. All were male. Two patients died (but not in relation to the treatment applied), while the fistula closed with conservative treatment at various time intervals from 15 to 80 days.

Rivo et al. achieved fistula closure in seven (87.5%) of the eight patients using sclerosant injection (ethanolamine or lauromacrogol 400) performed under general anesthesia [25]. All patients had developed bronchopleural fistula after lung resections as evidenced by the air leak in a thoracic drain and radiologic changes and confirmed by flexible bronchoscopy. In addition to sclerosant injection, patients received pleural drainage (open or closed thoracostomy) and antibiotics.

Stratakos et al. used silver nitrate in patients with BPF measuring 5 mm or less [26]. Through a flexible videobronchoscopy, they passed a standard bronchoscopic cytology brush covered with silver nitrate that was rubbed against the fistula's orifice, producing blanching and edema on the mucosa. They repeated the procedure until they obtained fistula closure or there was no tissue response after two bronchoscopic sessions that was considered a treatment failure. A total of 11 patients were treated with silver nitrate, and treatment success was achieved in 9, with no relapse after 11 months. A 60-year-old man with a right pneumothorax with severe respiratory distress caused by a persistent peripheral BPF was successfully treated with silver nitrate after failed conservative management [27] .

Ishikawa reported treating three BPF (5–6 mm in diameter) with a fibrin glue-coated collagen patch (FGCCP) and fibrin glue (FG) [28]. The first one was a

58-year-old man diagnosed with a 5 mm BPF 33 days after right middle and lower lobectomy. The second BPF measured 6 mm in a 61-year-old man and diagnosed after right pneumonectomy, while the third was a 67-year-old man presenting on the 11th day after right lower lobectomy. The FGCCP fragment was held in place for a minute, which is sufficient time for the FGCCP to stick, and the patch fragment was released. This is followed by direct application of FG using a two-channel catheter. While two patients required two treatments, the patient who had right lower lobectomy, and all were cured.

Gaspard et al. reported the use of endobronchial valves (EBV) in six patients with bronchopleural fistula [29]. The one-way valves were originally designed for the reduction in lung volume in patients with chronic obstructive pulmonary disease, and their anesthetic management is discussed in detail [30]. These valves are designed to allow air to exit, but not to enter, their subtended segments. It is suggested that EBV deployment should be considered for patients with BPF lasting 5 days despite appropriate management. It is also recommended to initially inflate an occlusive balloon is used (in the main bronchus followed by lobar and then segmental airways) to observe a decrease in rate of air leak through the water chamber of a water seal chest drain, allowing for five breathing cycles. If the desired results are obtained and the patient is persistently stable, either the chest tube is removed or a Heimlich valve is attached to the chest tube. The EBVs themselves are removed bronchoscopically approximately 6 weeks after insertion.

Both dedicated (customized) and modified existing stents are also used in the treatment of BPF [31]. In a single center, 148 patients with BPF were successfully treated with occlusive stents, of which 143/148 (96.6%) were treated with a single treatment and the remainder after two attempts.

In a single center, 30 patients (11 females vs. 19 males; mean age 48.03 ± 20.33 years) with BPF were treated (between 2018 and 2024) with Vaseline gauze, shape-adjustable silicone plug, sutured silicone tube, or covered metallic stent. Similar approaches are employed by other clinicians [11]. Yet more options for BPF closure are cardiac septal occluders, and endobronchial Watanabe spigots and future developments might include mesenchymal stem cells and three-dimensional (3D)-printed stents [22].

9.3 Anesthesia Management

9.3.1 Preprocedure Evaluation

The American College of Chest Physicians recommends intervention if the leak persists >4 days. It should be clear from the preceding discussion that the majority of patients presenting for bronchoscopic management of BPF are likely to be in poor general condition. This is related to both the pathology that has led to the fistula and its treatment—typically pneumonectomy or a lobectomy. Those who developed BPF after pneumonectomy are likely to be sicker than those who underwent lobectomy. The patients are likely to have lost weight, have a pleural drain, possibly septic, and short of breath. If the cause for fistula is lung cancer (a common reason for lung resections), there could be a long-standing history of smoking and associated COPD. Of course, not all BPFs are related to lung resection. Trauma (open or closed chest injury), lung abscess, empyema, bronchiectasis, and tuberculosis are other causes, and the general condition of the patient is likely to be, at least partially, related to them.

Dinesh et al. reported a case of BPF presenting as primary spontaneous right pneumothorax with severe respiratory distress. The patient had an intercostal drain with underwater seal that was inserted from the left fifth intercostal space in the midaxillary line [27]. Methylene blue might be injected through the intercostal tube to locate the site of BPF. Rarely, a bronchopleural fistula may present with diffuse swelling and crepitus of the face, chest, and extremities due to subcutaneous air [32]. In this patient, a CT scan of the chest showed a tumor in the left lung with associated pneumothorax, extensive subcutaneous emphysema, and pneumomediastinum throughout the thorax. Other presentations include life-threatening airway obstruction (due to subcutaneous emphysema) that must be emergently treated with endotracheal intubation [33]. Clinical presentation is usually subacute; however, it could be acute, presenting with sudden expectoration of potentially infected material from the pleural space due to airway communication [34].

In view of frequent preexisting pulmonary pathology, during preprocedure evaluation, it is important to focus on secondary cardiac complications, including pulmonary hypertension and right ventricular dysfunction.

Clinically, one would expect low oxygen saturation depending on the amount of lost air exchange area. The loss is related to many factors such as surgery (pneumonectomy/lobectomy of one or more lobes), compression of the normal lung, and pneumonia in the remainder of the lung/lungs. Arterial blood gas might show hypoxemia, hypercapnia, and acidosis (respiratory or combined). There is likely to be continuous loss of inspired gas from the fistula site, and, as a result, expired tidal volumes are bound to be smaller than inspired.

9.3.2 Airway, Monitoring, and Anesthesia Choice

In addition to the standard anesthesia goals, the specific challenges exist. In anesthetizing a patient presenting for surgical closure of a BPF, presence of a leak and potential retrograde soiling of potentially healthy lung is a major concern. Given the leak from the diseased lung into the pleural cavity, ventilation will be challenging. As a result, some form of lung isolation is essential. This applies to nonthoracic surgical procedures too [35]. However, the challenges are different for endoscopic closure. Losing the ventilation through the fistula is usually not a concern.

Induction is usually intravenous if necessary rapid sequence. Muscle relaxant with controlled ventilation is essential. A single lumen endotracheal tube is employed and positioned as per the desire of the pulmonologist. At the Jefferson University Hospital, Philadelphia, PA, USA, patients with BPF are brought into the bronchoscopy procedure room (out of operating room location) for evaluation as to the suitability of endobronchial valve placement. Initially, the pulmonologist attempts to isolate the segment where the leak is coming from using the sequential balloon occlusion technique. The aim is to achieve complete cessation of leak in the water chamber when the segment leading to the BPF is occluded by the balloon. We might not achieve this if there are multiple defects and/or collateral ventilation exists between segments/lobes. This isolation of segment is done before other treatment options like fibrin glue/sclerosants, etc., are employed. Occasionally, if a leak cannot be detected with adequate positive pressure ventilation, the anesthesia provider, the pulmonologist requests to increase the tidal volumes, provide a large volume manual breath, or administer PEEP. These maneuvers might elicit the leak. This is quite the opposite of what is done in bronchoscopic lung volume reduction procedures. If all the above maneuvers fail to elicit the leak and find the fistula, methylene blue is injected sequentially in the appropriate segments and observe the chest tube if the dye appears after each injection.

Monitoring is as per the American Society of Anesthesia minimum monitoring. However, additional monitoring may be needed in specific situations and patient populations.

9.4 Communications Between Airway and Viscera

These include tracheoesophageal fistula (TEF), bronchoesophageal fistula, gastrobronchial fistula, gastrotracheal fistula, bronchobiliary fistula, and colobronchial fistula. Recurrent chest infections and shortness of breath are some of the common symptoms. Being the most common, our discussion will mainly involve TEF. However, the term OEF is also used broadly to include all communications between airway (any location) and the esophagus.

9.4.1 Causes and Mechanisms

Airway involvement is common in esophageal cancer. Extrapulmonary malignant central airway obstruction is most commonly caused by esophageal cancer (EC) [36]. In a retrospective analysis of 804 patients with a diagnosis of EC, Goh et al. documented a 36.6% and 13.1% incidence of airway involvement and TEF [37]. Some of the predictors of airway involvement were location of the tumor (higher with midesophageal and upper esophageal), previous treatment with esophageal stenting, and chemotherapy or radiotherapy. In those who had TEF, survival was better with chemotherapy and combined airway and esophageal stenting.

In another retrospective analysis of 122 consecutive patients with EC, tumor location within 20 mm of the carina, prior radiotherapy, and/or esophageal stenting were significantly associated with the formation of TEF [38]. Tumor in the midesophagus or presence of TEF indicated poor survival. Similar to the study cited above, getting chemotherapy or esophageal stenting whether before or after airway intervention had better survival.

Other causes of TEF include infections, inhalation injuries, and traumatic damage [39]. Of the nonmalignant causes, endotracheal cuff-related trauma, usually related to prolonged mechanical ventilation, contributes to more than 75% [40]. Approximately 0.3–3% of ventilated patients end up with secondary erosion of the tracheal and esophageal walls [41].

The site of TEF is variable. While reviewing 207 patient records with TEF, Burt et al. found them in the following locations: trachea in 110 (53%), left main bronchus in 46 (22%), right bronchus in 33 (16%), lung parenchyma in 13 (6%), and multiple sites in 5 (2%) [42]. In terms of clinical presentations of malignant esophagorespiratory fistula, the following were noted: cough in 116 (56%), aspiration in 77 (37%), fever in 52 (25%), dysphagia in 39 (19%), pneumonia in 11 (5%), hemoptysis in 10 (5%), and chest pain in 10 (5%).

Both esophageal and bronchial malignancies can cause bronchoesophageal fistula (BEF) [43]. Among the non-malignant causes are infections such as tuberculosis, histoplasmosis, and actinomycosis. Heterotopic gastric mucosa in the midesophagus is another rare cause [44–48].

Gastrobronchial fistula (GBF) usually develops either early or late after esophagectomy with gastric pull-up and can occur anywhere in the respiratory tract, from the trachea to the lobar bronchus [49]. In an analysis of 24 studies (89 patients), Wang et al. found that cough was the main clinical presentation of thoracogastric airway fistula (TGAF), and the main bronchus was the most common place [50].

Information on gastrotracheal fistula is mostly in case reports. Nardella et al. discussed a case of gastrotracheal fistula following esophagectomy for cancer [51]. In this case, the patient was a 58-year-old man with distal third uT3N1 carcinoma of the esophagus that was removed (esophago-gastrectomy) followed by reconstruction by gastric pull-up. Fifteen days later, he developed severe bilateral basal pneumonia due to a necrotic defect 5 cm above the carina seen on a bronchoscopy. However, he was successfully managed with a covered stent in the trachea, along with clipping and glueing of the gastric fistular orifice. Nevertheless, the fistula recurred after 2 weeks requiring surgical intervention.

9.4.2 Nonsurgical Interventional Management

Self-expanding metal stents, degradable stents, silicone stents, fibrin glue injections, unidirectional umbrella valves in the bronchi, and congenital heart disease occluders are some of the options available to close the fistulae. Fibrin glue injections may be suitable for treating only small fistula (< 5 mm) [52].

Zhan et al. performed a single-center, retrospective study of malignant central airway obstruction (CAO) or tracheoesophageal fistula (TEF) receiving self-expanding metallic stent (SEMS) placement [53]. A total of 24 patients received SEMS for TEF. Also, 50% of patients with TEF showed improvement in their symptoms and the 3-month survival rate was low at 67%. Blackmon et al. reviewed 25 patients with esophageal or gastric leaks who were evaluated for stenting as primary treatment [54]. Of the 25 patients, 23 were managed with endoscopic stenting as primary treatment. Four patients presented with TEF: one as a complication of laryngectomy, or second from radiation and chemotherapy for lung cancer, and two from prolonged intubation. Of these, effective sealing was achieved in two patients. However, a case of TEF resulting from SEMS places in the esophagus to treat repeated strictures at the esophagogastric anastomosis after esophagectomy for an adenocarcinoma of distal esophagus is also reported [55].

9.5 Anesthesia Management

9.5.1 Preprocedure Assessment

TEF is an abnormal connection, typically between the esophagus and trachea or bronchi. Tracheal (or bronchial) and esophageal cancers and their treatment (surgery, radiotherapy, chemotherapy) are common causes. About 1 percent of patients with bronchogenic carcinoma and 5–15% of patients with esophageal cancer develop TEF [46, 56, 57]. Prolonged endotracheal intubation, trauma, and granulomatous infections like tuberculosis are other causes [52]. Overall, about half of all TEFs are acquired [58].

Complaints of dysphagia, persistent coughing (mainly after eating and drinking), weight loss, and pneumonia are frequent. Dyspnea, rarely hemoptysis, and pulmonary aspiration are other possible symptoms. Room air oxygen saturations could be low, and patients could be on supplemental oxygen. Ventilation in the ICU could be challenging [59]. The severity of the symptoms depends on the location and size of the fistulous opening. Most patients die within 3 months of fistula formation.

It is always a good practice to review findings of chest X-ray and CT scan with the pulmonologist and discuss the anesthesia plan. It is not uncommon to manage these fistulas with esophageal or both (tracheal-esophageal) stents, using either rigid or flexible bronchoscopy, with or without fluoroscopy [60]. These stents might allow improvement in health status in terms of weight gain and allow radiation treatment, or they could be purely palliative.

9.5.2 Airway, Monitoring, and Anesthesia Choice

Anesthesia and airway management for the treatment of TEF are extensively discussed in the literature [59, 61–65]. Although some are related to surgical management, the broad principles of airway management remain similar.

Dechong et al. performed a single-center study between July 2020 and July 2023 and reviewed 34 anesthesia records for endoscopic TEF occlusion [62]. Their airway management consisted of nasal catheter oxygen ($n = 5$), high-flow nasal cannula oxygen therapy ($n = 4$), and tracheal intubation ($n = 25$). Using a 5.5-mm endotracheal tube (ETT) provided better procedure conditions than the other two options that required significantly longer surgical times. Local anesthetic aerosol inhalation was used in all patients. To minimize the risk of aspiration, they performed an unseated gastroscopy before tracheal intubation. Culturally, it may be difficult to convince patients for such awake gastroscopy in the USA. The ETT was positioned above the carina, so that the distal part of the cuff is below the fistula. The distance between the fistula and the carina was 3–5 cm. They used propofol and remifentanil for induction and rocuronium to facilitate intubation. One patient had a preexisting tracheostomy stoma. Anesthesia was maintained either with intravenous drug infusions or inhalational agents. The procedure of occluder implantation included combined gastroscopy and tracheoscopy, with implant being placed into the fistula through endoscopic forceps under direct vision of the gastroscope. Biopsy forceps passed under bronchoscopic vision facilitated the release of the occluder on the tracheal side. They confirmed occlusion on both tracheal and esophageal ends and sprayed 0.2% methylene blue on the fistula opening on the gastroscope side to observe leak and determine the successful occlusion.

Chiartas et al. deliberately performed a tight-sided endobronchial intubation (guided by a fiberoptic bronchoscope) to treat the leak that was happening with endotracheal placement [59]. A patient who developed TEF from a tracheal stent that was placed to treat tracheal stenosis was similarly managed with an endobronchial tube by Ashraf et al. [61]. Huang used an inner diameter 5.5 mm ETT for managing the airway and providing general anesthesia to place a gastrointestinal occluder device [65].

At the Thomas Jefferson University Hospital, Philadelphia, PA, USA, they undertake a combined procedure between interventional pulmonology and advanced gastrointestinal (GI) endoscopy teams. The decision of airway stenting preceding the GI stent is done on a case-by-case basis based on the location/s of the tracheo-esophageal fistula. Factors such as preexisting airway obstruction from the tumor (as noted in the CT scan) anticipated difficulty or incomplete closure by the GI stent. In general, the teams would prefer to avoid double stenting in malignant cases as the radial pressure exerted by the self-expanding metallic stents in opposing directions can potentially keep the fistula open/worsen it. Some of the reasons where airway stenting is considered after placement of GI stent are evidence of ongoing aspiration events clinically or as evidenced by barium swallow study.

In general, for BPF, at our hospital, the pulmonologist attempts to quantify the leak. A grading of leak is performed based on the number of chamber leak, whether leak is on inspiration/expiration or continuous. Specialized devices and pleural manometry are available to measure the actual volume of TV lost during each breath.

In some cases (e.g., ventilated patients), newer ventilators can automatically calculate the leak. While treating BPF/TEF in ventilated patients, conservative management such as zero peep and quick weaning from positive pressure ventilation is an option.

References

1. Fistula - an overview | ScienceDirect Topics [Internet]. [cited 2025 Mar 31]. Available from: https://www.sciencedirect.com/topics/medicine-and-dentistry/fistula
2. Aliaga F, Grosu HB, Vial MR. Overview of Bronchopleural fistula management, with a focus on Bronchoscopic treatment. Curr Pulmonol Rep. 2022;11(2):65–73.
3. Dezube AR, Dolan DP, Mazzola E, Kucukak S, De Leon LE, Bueno R, et al. Risk factors for prolonged air leak and need for intervention following lung resection. Interact Cardiovasc Thorac Surg. 2021;34(2):212–8.
4. Clark JM, Cooke DT, Brown LM. Management of complications after lung resection: prolonged air leak and bronchopleural fistula. Thorac Surg Clin. 2020;30(3):347–58.
5. Mueller MR, Marzluf BA. The anticipation and management of air leaks and residual spaces post lung resection. J Thorac Dis. 2014;6(3):271–84.
6. Sirbu H, Busch T, Aleksic I, Schreiner W, Oster O, Dalichau H. Bronchopleural fistula in the surgery of non-small cell lung cancer: incidence, risk factors, and management. Ann Thorac Cardiovasc Surg. 2001;7(6):330–6.
7. Birdas TJ, Morad MH, Okereke IC, Rieger KM, Kruter LE, Mathur PN, et al. Risk factors for bronchopleural fistula after right pneumonectomy: does eliminating the stump diverticulum provide protection. Ann Surg Oncol. 2012;19(4):1336–42.
8. Panagopoulos ND, Apostolakis E, Koletsis E, Prokakis C, Hountis P, Sakellaropoulos G, et al. Low incidence of bronchopleural fistula after pneumonectomy for lung cancer. Interact Cardiovasc Thorac Surg. 2009;9(4):571–5.
9. Forde PM, Spicer J, Lu S, Provencio M, Mitsudomi T, Awad MM, et al. Neoadjuvant nivolumab plus chemotherapy in resectable lung cancer. N Engl J Med. 2022;386(21):1973–85.
10. Alpert JB, Godoy MCB, Degroot PM, Truong MT, Ko JP. Imaging the post-thoracotomy patient: anatomic changes and postoperative complications. Radiol Clin North Am. 2014;52(1):85–103.
11. Lois M, Noppen M. Bronchopleural fistulas: an overview of the problem with special focus on endoscopic management. Chest. 2005;128(6):3955–65.
12. Hsieh YC, Wang CW, Lai SH, Lai JY, Wong KS, Huang YC, et al. Necrotizing pneumococcal pneumonia with bronchopleural fistula among children in Taiwan. Pediatr Infect Dis J. 2011;30(9):740–4.
13. Sekarsari D, Handoyo S, Amal MY, Kharismarini P. Necrotizing pneumonia with bronchopleural fistula as an uncommon complication of pneumonia in children: a case report. Radiol Case Rep. 2021;16(8):2077–80.
14. Widysanto A, Liem M, Puspita KD, Pradhana CML. Management of necrotizing pneumonia with bronchopleural fistula caused by multidrug-resistant Acinetobacter baumannii. Respirol Case Rep. 2020;8(8):e00662.
15. Fraga JC, Holanda FC, Silva NZ, Oliveira MF, Isolan PS, Procianoy EF. Bronchopleural fistula following COVID-19 and necrotizing pneumonia in childhood: treatment with intrapleural vacuum-assisted closure therapy. Respirol Case Rep. 2025;13(3):e70134.
16. Hosna AU, Miller D. A case of bronchopleural fistula and hydropneumothorax in a patient with necrotizing pneumonia complicated by Mycobacterium avium complex. Cureus. 14(10):e30280.
17. Ravikanth R, Mathew S, Pinto DS. Management of acquired bronchopleural fistula due to chemical pneumonia. Tzu-Chi Med J. 2018;30(2):116–8.
18. Matsunaga T, Suzuki K, Hattori A, Fukui M, Takamochi K. Risk factors for bronchopleural fistula based on surgical procedure and sex in 4794 consecutive patients undergoing anatomical pulmonary resection. Surg Today. 2024;54(6):617–26.
19. Woldemariam ST, Molla IB, Merine SK, Yilma DG. Prevalence and treatment outcome of bronchopleural fistula: a multi-center study in Ethiopia. J Cardiothorac Surg. 2023;18(1):227.
20. Tsubakimoto M, Murayama S, Iraha R, Kamiya H, Tsuchiya N, Yamashiro T. Can peripheral bronchopleural fistula demonstrated on computed tomography be treated conservatively? A retrospective analysis. J Comput Assist Tomogr. 2016;40(1):86–90.

21. Egyud M, Suzuki K. Post-resection complications: abscesses, empyemas, bronchopleural fistulas. J Thorac Dis. 2018;10(Suppl 28):S3408–18.
22. Jin L, Li Y. Bronchoscopic interventions for bronchopleural fistulas. Ther Adv Respir Dis. 2023;17:17534666231164541.
23. Boudaya MS, Smadhi H, Zribi H, Mohamed J, Ammar J, Mestiri T, et al. Conservative management of postoperative bronchopleural fistulas. J Thorac Cardiovasc Surg. 2013;146(3):575–9.
24. Naranjo Gómez JM, Carbajo Carbajo M, Valdivia Concha D, Campo-Cañaveral de la Cruz JL. Conservative treatment of post-lobectomy bronchopleural fistula. Interact Cardiovasc Thorac Surg. 2012;15(1):152–4.
25. Rivo E, Quiroga J, García-Prim JM, Obeso A, Soro J, Oseira A, et al. Bronchoscopic sclerosis of post-resectional bronchial fistulas. Asian Cardiovasc Thorac Ann. 2019;27(2):93–7.
26. Stratakos G, Zuccatosta L, Porfyridis I, Sediari M, Zisis C, Mariatou V, et al. Silver nitrate through flexible bronchoscope in the treatment of bronchopleural fistulae. J Thorac Cardiovasc Surg. 2009;138(3):603–7.
27. Mehta D, Mehta C, Wadhwa S, Bassi SD, Verma M, Singla S. Silver nitrate in interventional pulmonology: treating a case of persistent bronchopleural fistula. J Bronchol Interv Pulmonol. 2011;18(2):184.
28. Ishikawa K, Kato T, Aragaki M, Hase R, Saikai T, Matsui Y, et al. Endobronchial closure of a bronchopleural fistula using a fibrin glue-coated collagen patch and fibrin glue. Ann Thorac Cardiovasc Surg Off J Assoc Thorac Cardiovasc Surg Asia. 2013;19(6):423–7.
29. Gaspard D, Bartter T, Boujaoude Z, Raja H, Arya R, Meena N, et al. Endobronchial valves for bronchopleural fistula: pitfalls and principles. Ther Adv Respir Dis. 2017;11(1):3–8.
30. Goudra B, Sundararaman L, Chandar P, Green M. Anesthesia for bronchoscopy-an update. J Clin Med. 2024;13(21):6471.
31. Han X, Yin M, Li L, Zhu M, Ren K, Qi Y, et al. Customized airway stenting for bronchopleural fistula after pulmonary resection by interventional technique: single-center study of 148 consecutive patients. Surg Endosc. 2018;32(10):4116–24.
32. Liang J, Field A, Liang K. Bronchopleural fistula. West J Emerg Med. 2013;14(5):409–10.
33. Gibney RT, Finnegan B, FitzGerald MX, Lynch V. Upper airway obstruction caused by massive subcutaneous emphysema. Intensive Care Med. 1984;10(1):43–4.
34. Høier-Madsen K, Schulze, Svend, Pedersen, Vilhelm Møller, Halkier E. Management of bronchopleural fistula following pneumonectomy. Scand J Thorac Cardiovasc Surg. 1984;18(3):263–6.
35. Garrett AL, Carrizal MC, Weber LV, Turner KR, Patel RS, Meyers LD. Anesthetic management of a bronchopleural fistula for non-thoracic surgery. J Cardiothorac Vasc Anesth [Internet]. 2024 [cited 2025 Apr 8]; Available from: https://www.sciencedirect.com/science/article/pii/S1053077024005184
36. Niwas R, Chawla G, Chauhan NK, Dutt N. Esophageal cancer, central airway obstruction, and lots more: a collaborative approach to a challenging scenario. Turk Thorac J. 2021;22(2):175–8.
37. Goh KJ, Lee P, Foo AZX, Tan EH, Ong HS, Hsu AAL. Characteristics and outcomes of airway involvement in esophageal cancer. Ann Thorac Surg. 2021;112(3):912–20.
38. Leong CKL, Foo AZX, Goh KJ, Hsu AAL, Ho AR, Ng MCH, et al. Airway interventions for tracheobronchial involvement in esophageal carcinoma: a retrospective cohort outcome study and algorithmic approach. J Thorac Dis. 2022;14(7):2565–78.
39. Kim HS, Khemasuwan D, Diaz-Mendoza J, Mehta AC. Management of tracheo-oesophageal fistula in adults. Eur Respir Rev [Internet]. 2020 [cited 2025 Apr 8];29(158). Available from: https://publications.ersnet.org/content/errev/29/158/200094
40. Diddee R, Shaw IH. Acquired tracheo-oesophageal fistula in adults. Contin Educ Anaesth Crit Care Pain. 2006;6(3):105–8.
41. Couraud L, Ballester MJ, Delaisement C. Acquired tracheoesophageal fistula and its management. Semin Thorac Cardiovasc Surg. 1996;8(4):392–9.
42. Burt M, Diehl W, Martini N, Bains MS, Ginsberg RJ, McCormack PM, et al. Malignant esophagorespiratory fistula: management options and survival. Ann Thorac Surg. 1991;52(6):1222–9.
43. Argüder E, Aykun G, Karalezli A, Hasanoglu HC. Bronchoesophageal fistula. J Bronchol Interv Pulmonol. 2012;19(1):47.

44. Kleinberg LR, Brock MV, Jagannath SB, Abelof MD, Armitage JO, Niederhuber JE, et al. Cancer of the esophagus. In: Abeloff's clinical oncology. Philadelphia, PA: Churchill Livingstone, An Imprint of Elsevier; 2008. p. 1399–429.
45. Martini N, Goodner JT, D'Angio GJ, et al. Tracheoesophageal fistula due to cancer. J Thorac Cardiovasc Surg. 1970;59:319–24.
46. Shin JH, Song HY, Ko GY, et al. Esophagorespiratory fistula: long-term results of palliative treatment with covered expandable metallic stents in 61 patients. Radiology. 2004;232:252–9.
47. Spalding AR, Burney DP, Richie RE. Acquired benign bronchoesophageal fistulas in the adult. Ann Thorac Surg. 1979;28:378–83.
48. Risher WH, Arensman RM, Ochsner JL. Congenital bronchoesophageal fistula. Ann Thorac Surg. 1990;49:500–5.
49. Wang SY, Yuan WC, Wu EB. Airway management during left-sided gastrobronchial fistula repair after esophagectomy for esophageal carcinoma: a case report. Medicine (Baltimore). 2021;100(35):e27133.
50. Li Y, Wang Y, Chen J, Li Z, Liu J, Zhou X, et al. Management of thoracogastric airway fistula after esophagectomy for esophageal cancer: a systematic literature review. J Int Med Res. 2020;48(5):0300060520926025.
51. Nardella JE, Van Raemdonck D, Piessevaux H, Deprez P, Droissart R, Staudt JP, et al. Gastro-tracheal fistula - unusual and life threatening complication after esophagectomy for cancer: a case report. J Cardiothorac Surg. 2009;4:69.
52. Shah SJ, Jadhav UE, Agrawal DP. Acquired tracheo-esophageal fistula in adult—a classical case of 'what not to do' Indian J Thorac Cardiovasc Surg 2022;38(4):442–4.
53. Bai Y, Zhan K, Chi J, Jiang J, Li S, Yin Y, et al. Self-expandable metal stent in the management of malignant airway disorders. Front Med. 2022;9:902488.
54. Blackmon SH, Santora R, Schwarz P, Barroso A, Dunkin BJ. Utility of removable esophageal covered self-expanding metal stents for leak and fistula management. Ann Thorac Surg. 2010;89(3):931–6; discussion 936–937
55. Schowengerdt CG. Tracheoesophageal fistula caused by a self-expanding esophageal stent. Ann Thorac Surg. 1999;67(3):830–1.
56. Chen YH, Li SH, Chiu YC, Lu HI, Huang CH, Rau KM, et al. Comparative study of esophageal stent and feeding gastrostomy/jejunostomy for tracheoesophageal fistula caused by esophageal squamous cell carcinoma. PLoS One. 2012;7(8):e42766.
57. Balazs A, Kupcsulik PK, Galambos Z. Esophagorespiratory fistulas of tumorous origin. Non-operative management of 264 cases in a 20-year period. Eur J Cardio-Thorac Surg Off J Eur Assoc Cardio-Thorac Surg. 2008;34(5):1103–7.
58. Reed MF, Mathisen DJ. Tracheoesophageal fistula. Chest Surg Clin N Am. 2003;13:271–89.
59. Chiartas EJ, Neurock J, Rubin K. Tracheoesophageal fistula: airway management and temporization in a community hospital setting. Cureus. 15(3):e35838.
60. Stratakos G, Zisis C, Bellenis I, Filaditaki V, Liapikou A, Zakynthinos S, et al. Tracheoesophageal fistula managed with tracheal stent through flexible bronchoscopy without fluoroscopy. Monaldi Arch Chest Dis. 2006;65(4):225–7.
61. Ashraf U, Farooq O, Ashfaq AD, Butt F, Khattak S. Airway management of a patient with tracheoesophageal fistula and tracheal stent. Cureus. 14(10):e30524.
62. Dechong Z, He H, Jigang Z, Cunming L. Airway and anesthesia management in tracheo-esophageal fistula closure implantation: a single-centre retrospective study. J Cardiothorac Surg. 2024;19(1):172.
63. Au CL, White SA, Grant RP. A novel intubation technique for tracheoesophageal fistula in adults. Can J Anaesth. 1999;46(7):688–91.
64. Wang L, Chen F. Anesthetic consideration of a patient with acquired tracheoesophageal fistula undergoing radical left colectomy for sigmoid cancer. Quant Imaging Med Surg. 2024;14(7):5273–6.
65. Huang H, Zhang J, Li L, Zhang G, Zhu D. Anesthesia management for tracheoesophageal fistula closed with a new gastrointestinal occluder device: a case report. J Cardiothorac Surg. 2022;17(1):287.

Anesthesia for Placement of Endobronchial Valves

10

Labib Mahmoud

10.1 Introduction

Endobronchial valves (EBVs) are innovative, minimally invasive devices used in the management of severe emphysema, a subset of chronic obstructive pulmonary disease (COPD) [1]. These one-way valves facilitate the evacuation of air from hyperinflated lung segments while preventing air re-entry, thereby reducing lung hyperinflation, improving lung mechanics, and enhancing patient quality of life [2]. COPD is a major cause of morbidity and mortality worldwide, with severe emphysema representing a particularly debilitating form. According to the World Health Organization (2021), COPD is the third leading cause of death globally, responsible for approximately three million deaths annually [3].

EBVs have emerged as a viable alternative to more invasive surgical options, such as lung volume reduction surgery (LVRS) and lung transplantation [4]. The development and evolution of EBVs have been driven by the need to provide effective treatment options that can improve lung function and quality of life while minimizing the risks associated with more invasive procedures. The mechanism of action involves the selective placement of valves in airways leading to diseased lung segments, creating a controlled collapse of these segments and improving the overall mechanics of the remaining healthier lung tissue [2].

This chapter will discuss the indications, clinical studies, patient risk stratification, preoperative optimization, intraoperative management, postoperative complications, and special situations related to anesthesia for EBV placement.

L. Mahmoud (✉)
Henry Ford Hospital, Detroit, MI, USA
e-mail: ldebian1@hfhs.org

M. Sarkiss (ed.), *Anesthesia for Interventional Pulmonary Procedures*,
https://doi.org/10.1007/978-3-032-12007-6_10

10.2 Indications

EBV placement is primarily indicated for patients with severe emphysema characterized by substantial hyperinflation and air trapping who have not adequately responded to conventional medical treatments and are not suitable candidates for surgical lung volume reduction (LVRS) or lung transplantation. Specific selection criteria include

- Severe airflow obstruction: post-bronchodilator forced expiratory volume in 1 second (FEV1) between 15% and 45% of predicted [4].
- Significant hyperinflation: total lung capacity (TLC) greater than 100% of predicted [4].
- Marked air trapping: residual volume (RV) greater than or equal to 175% of predicted [4].
- Heterogeneous disease pattern: target lobe with at least 50% destruction and an absolute difference of $\geq$15 in destruction scores between the targeted and ipsilateral lobes, as determined by quantitative computed tomography (CT) analysis [2].

10.3 Contraindications

- Collateral ventilation (CV): the presence of collateral ventilation between the target lobe and adjacent lobes, as assessed by the Chartis system, can lead to treatment failure [5].
- Other contraindications: severe comorbidities, active infections, or inadequate fissure integrity that would preclude effective lung deflation [6].

10.4 Patient Evaluation Process

In addition to the primary criteria, patients must undergo a comprehensive evaluation to determine their overall health status and suitability for EBV placement. This includes a detailed medical history, physical examination, and a series of diagnostic tests. Imaging studies, such as high-resolution computed tomography (CT) scans, play a critical role in assessing the extent of emphysema and identifying suitable target lobes for valve placement. Pulmonary function tests (PFTs) are essential to evaluate the severity of airflow obstruction and hyperinflation. Cardiopulmonary exercise testing may also be performed to assess exercise tolerance and identify any cardiovascular limitations.

Patients who are current smokers must be enrolled in smoking cessation programs as continued smoking can significantly reduce the effectiveness of EBVs and increase the risk of complications. Nutritional status is another important consideration as malnutrition is common in advanced COPD and can negatively impact recovery. Patients with a body mass index (BMI) less than 20 kg/m^2 may require nutritional supplementation and support. In summary

- *Multidisciplinary team involvement:* a team comprising *pulmonologists, radiologists, and thoracic surgeons* collaborates to ensure appropriate patient selection and procedural planning [1].
- *Comprehensive assessment:* detailed *medical history, physical examination, and diagnostic tests*, including *high-resolution CT scans and pulmonary function tests*, are essential to evaluate disease severity and suitability for EBV placement [2].
- *Smoking cessation:* patients must be enrolled in *smoking cessation programs*, as continued smoking can significantly reduce the effectiveness of EBVs and increase the risk of complications [1].
- *Nutritional status:* assessment and *optimization of nutritional status* are important, as *malnutrition* is common in advanced COPD and can negatively impact recovery [6].

10.4.1 Overview of Main Clinical Studies

Several pivotal studies have underpinned the clinical adoption of EBVs in the treatment of emphysema:

1. *The VENT Study (2006):* A landmark randomized controlled trial (RCT) demonstrating significant improvements in lung function, exercise capacity, and quality of life in patients receiving EBVs compared to those receiving standard medical care. The study included 321 patients, and those in the EBV group showed a 6.8% improvement in FEV1 and a 9.3-meter increase in the 6-minute walk distance (6MWD) [2].
2. *The TRANSFORM Study (2017):* Focused on patients with heterogeneous emphysema. In a randomized study, 65 subjects receiving endobronchial valve (EBV) therapy showed significantly better outcomes compared to 32 subjects receiving standard care. At 6 months, 56.3% of the EBV group achieved an FEV1 improvement of 12% or more compared to just 3.2% in the standard care group ($P < 0.001$). The EBV group also demonstrated a significant reduction in residual volume and improvements in 6-minute walk distance, St. George's Respiratory Questionnaire score, and BODE index, highlighting the therapy's effectiveness in enhancing lung function and exercise capacity. Pneumothorax was the most common adverse event, affecting 29.2% of EBV subjects [5].
3. *The LIBERATE Study (2018):* In a study with 190 subjects (128 receiving endobronchial valve [EBV] therapy and 62 receiving standard of care [SoC]), 47.7% of the EBV group achieved a 15% or greater improvement in FEV1 at 12 months compared to 16.8% in the SoC group ($P < 0.001$). The EBV group also showed significant improvements in FEV1, 6-minute walk distance, and quality of life (SGRQ score) compared to SoC. Reductions in hyperinflation and dyspnea were also noted in the EBV group. Pneumothorax was the most common serious adverse event, occurring in 26.6% of EBV subjects, with four deaths reported during the treatment period [4].

4. *The EMPROVE Study (2019)* evaluated the Spiration Valve System (SVS) versus medical management alone in patients with severe heterogeneous emphysema. At 6 months, the SVS significantly improved lung function (FEV_1 increased by 0.101 L) and secondary outcomes, including hyperinflation, dyspnea, and health status, but not the 6-minute walk distance. Serious thoracic adverse events, primarily pneumothorax, were more common in the SVS group (31.0% vs. 11.9%). The study concluded that SVS offers significant clinical benefits with an acceptable safety profile [7].

These studies collectively underscore the effectiveness of EBVs in improving clinical outcomes in selected patients with severe emphysema. However, it is important to acknowledge the limitations of these studies, including variations in patient populations, study designs, and outcome measures. Future research should focus on refining patient selection criteria, exploring the long-term effects of EBV treatment, and comparing EBVs with other emerging therapies for emphysema.

10.5 Patient Risk Stratification and Optimization Preoperatively

Successful EBV placement requires meticulous patient selection and preoperative optimization. Essential considerations include

- Pulmonary function testing: Detailed assessment to confirm the severity of emphysema and the extent of air trapping. This includes spirometry, body plethysmography, and diffusion capacity testing. Pulmonary function testing provides critical information about the patient's respiratory mechanics and gas exchange capabilities, which are essential for predicting the potential benefits and risks of EBV placement [4].
- Imaging studies: High-resolution CT scans to identify suitable target lobes for valve placement and to assess fissure completeness, which is crucial for predicting procedural success. Imaging studies provide detailed anatomical information, allowing for precise planning of the EBV placement [2]. The use of advanced imaging techniques, such as 3D reconstructions and quantitative CT analysis, can further enhance the accuracy of patient selection and procedure planning.
- Cardiovascular assessment: Given the high prevalence of comorbid cardiovascular diseases in this patient population, thorough evaluation, including echocardiography and stress testing, may be necessary [1]. This is essential to assess cardiac function and identify any underlying conditions that may need to be optimized before the procedure. Cardiovascular assessment helps identify patients at higher risk for perioperative complications and guides the management of comorbid conditions.
- Pulmonary hypertension considerations: Pulmonary hypertension (PH) is common in advanced emphysema and can complicate EBV placement. Patients

should be screened for PH using echocardiography, and those with significant PH may require additional optimization and monitoring [8]. The management of PH involves the use of vasodilators, diuretics, and careful fluid balance. It is crucial to ensure that PH is well-controlled before proceeding with the procedure. Optimizing PH can improve perioperative outcomes and reduce the risk of complications related to increased pulmonary vascular resistance.
- Nutritional status: Malnutrition is common in advanced COPD and should be addressed through dietary interventions and nutritional supplementation to improve overall health status preoperatively. Nutritional support can help enhance respiratory muscle strength and improve postoperative recovery. Nutritional assessment includes evaluating body mass index (BMI), muscle mass, and dietary intake. Interventions may include high-protein diets, nutritional supplements, and consultation with a dietitian.
- Smoking cessation: Essential for reducing perioperative complications and improving overall lung health. Patients should be enrolled in smoking cessation programs and provided with support to quit smoking [1]. Smoking cessation can significantly improve respiratory function, reduce the risk of infections, and enhance overall surgical outcomes.
- Management of comorbid conditions: Optimization of cardiovascular diseases, diabetes, and any ongoing infections is crucial to minimize perioperative risks [4]. This includes managing hypertension, controlling blood glucose levels, and treating any active infections. Comprehensive management of comorbidities involves a multidisciplinary approach, including primary care physicians, cardiologists, endocrinologists, and infectious disease specialists.

10.6 Intraoperative Management and Anesthetic Techniques

The placement of EBVs is typically performed under general anesthesia or deep sedation, depending on patient factors, procedural complexity, and interventional pulmonologist preferences. Key aspects of intraoperative management include

- *Airway management:* Securing the airway with endotracheal intubation or a laryngeal mask airway (LMA) is crucial to facilitate bronchoscopy and valve placement. Larger endotracheal tubes are generally advantageous as they provide better access and maneuverability for the bronchoscopic equipment, thereby facilitating the precise placement of the valves.
- *Ventilation strategies:* Careful management to avoid hyperinflation and barotrauma is essential. This includes using low tidal volumes (4–6 mL/kg of ideal body weight) and permissive hypercapnia strategies. Maintaining adequate oxygenation while preventing further lung damage is a critical balance. Ventilation strategies should be individualized based on the patient's baseline respiratory function and intraoperative response.
- *Hemodynamic monitoring:* Continuous monitoring of heart rate, blood pressure, and oxygen saturation. In high-risk patients, arterial line placement may be

warranted for continuous blood pressure monitoring and frequent blood gas analysis. This allows for real-time assessment of hemodynamic stability and respiratory function. Advanced hemodynamic monitoring, including cardiac output measurement and central venous pressure monitoring, may be considered in patients with significant cardiovascular comorbidities.

- *Anesthetic agents:* The use of short-acting agents such as propofol, remifentanil, and sevoflurane allows for rapid recovery post-procedure. These agents provide adequate sedation and analgesia while minimizing respiratory depression postoperatively. The choice of anesthetic agents should be tailored to the individual patient's needs and the duration of the procedure. The use of balanced anesthesia, combining multiple agents to achieve optimal sedation, analgesia, and muscle relaxation, can enhance the safety and efficacy of the procedure.
- *Bronchoscopic guidance:* Continuous coordination with the interventional pulmonologist during valve placement to ensure accurate positioning and deployment of EBVs. This involves real-time communication and collaboration to achieve optimal results. The use of advanced bronchoscopic techniques, such as fluoroscopic guidance and navigation bronchoscopy, can further improve the accuracy and success of EBV placement.

10.7 Postoperative Complications and Management

Postoperative care focuses on monitoring for and managing potential complications:

- Pneumothorax: A common complication following EBV therapy, occurring in up to 26.6% of patients [4]. Patients should be closely monitored with serial chest X-rays. Management may include observation for small pneumothoraces or chest tube placement for larger or symptomatic pneumothoraces. Early detection and prompt intervention are crucial to prevent deterioration. Preventive measures, such as avoiding excessive positive pressure ventilation and minimizing procedural trauma, can reduce the risk of pneumothorax.
- Infection: Prophylactic antibiotics may be considered to reduce the risk of acute exacerbations of COPD following EBV placement [9]. Vigilant monitoring for signs of pneumonia or other infections is essential. Patients should be educated on recognizing symptoms of infection and seeking timely medical attention. Postoperative care includes regular follow-up visits, sputum cultures, and appropriate antibiotic therapy based on microbiological findings.
- Valve migration: Although rare, valve migration or expectoration has been reported in approximately 2.1% of cases [10]. This may necessitate follow-up bronchoscopy for repositioning or removal of the valve. Regular follow-up appointments and imaging studies are essential to monitor valve position and function. Ensuring proper valve placement and secure deployment during the procedure can minimize the risk of migration.

- Exacerbation of COPD: COPD exacerbations have been reported post-EBV placement, with rates varying across studies. One study reported a 21.2% rate of acute exacerbations following bronchoscopic lung volume reduction with EBVs [9]. Prompt management with bronchodilators, steroids, and supportive care is essential. Patients should have a clear action plan for managing exacerbations and should be provided with appropriate medications. Long-term follow-up includes optimizing COPD management, regular pulmonary rehabilitation, and lifestyle modifications to prevent future exacerbations.

10.8 Special Situations

Certain clinical scenarios require tailored anesthetic and procedural approaches:

- Previous thoracic surgery: Scar tissue can complicate valve placement, requiring advanced imaging and careful procedural planning. Preoperative assessment should include detailed imaging studies, such as contrast-enhanced CT scans, to identify anatomical challenges and plan the procedure accordingly. Intraoperative strategies may include using flexible bronchoscopes and advanced navigation tools to maneuver through scarred area.
- Bullous emphysema: Patients with bullous disease have an increased risk of pneumothorax, necessitating meticulous technique and close postoperative monitoring [11]. In such cases, preoperative imaging is crucial to identify the location and extent of bullae. Intraoperative precautions include gentle handling of lung tissues and avoiding excessive positive pressure ventilation. Postoperative care involves vigilant monitoring for pneumothorax and prompt intervention if it occurs.
- Severe hypoxemia: Preoperative optimization with oxygen therapy and intraoperative strategies to maintain oxygenation are crucial [12]. High-flow nasal cannula (HFNC) or noninvasive ventilation (NIV) may be used postoperatively to support respiratory function. Intraoperative measures include optimizing lung ventilation-perfusion matching, using high-inspired oxygen concentrations, and applying positive end-expiratory pressure (PEEP) to prevent alveolar collapse.

10.8.1 Fissure Completion Surgery

In some cases, incomplete fissures may impede effective lung deflation with EBVs alone. Fissure completion surgery, involving either surgical or endoscopic techniques to complete the fissure, can enhance the effectiveness of EBVs [13]. This approach requires a multidisciplinary team and careful planning to balance the benefits of enhanced lung deflation against the risks of additional surgical intervention. Techniques include

1. *Surgical fissure completion:* Traditional thoracoscopic or open surgery to complete the fissure. This is more invasive but may be necessary in cases where endoscopic techniques are insufficient. Surgical completion involves creating a complete separation between lobes to prevent collateral ventilation. The procedure may include stapling or suturing the fissure and ensuring airtight closure.
2. *Endoscopic fissure completion:* Minimally invasive methods using endoscopic tools to complete the fissure, often performed in conjunction with EBV placement. Endoscopic techniques may involve the use of sealants, plugs, or energy-based devices to close incomplete fissures. These methods are less invasive than surgical approaches and can be performed during the same session as EBV placement.

10.9 Conclusion

Anesthesia for the placement of endobronchial valves requires a thorough understanding of the patient's respiratory and cardiovascular status, meticulous preoperative optimization, and careful intraoperative management. Adhering to established protocols and being prepared to manage complications, anesthesiologists play a crucial role in ensuring the safety and success of this innovative procedure. The multidisciplinary approach, involving collaboration between pulmonologists, anesthesiologists, radiologists, and surgeons, is essential for optimizing patient outcomes. As the field of interventional pulmonology continues to evolve, ongoing research and technological advancements will further enhance the effectiveness and safety of EBV placement for patients with severe emphysema.

References

1. Alshabani K, Gildea TR, Machuzak M, Cicenia J, Hatipoglu U. Bronchoscopic lung volume reduction with valves: what should the internist know? Cleve Clin J Med. 2020;87(5):278–87.
2. Sciurba FC, Ernst A, Herth FJ, Strange C, Criner GJ, Marquette CH, et al. A randomized study of endobronchial valves for advanced emphysema. N Engl J Med. 2010;363(13):1233–44.
3. Organization WH. COPD fact sheet. 2021.
4. Criner GJ, Sue R, Wright S, Dransfield M, Rivas-Perez H, Wiese T, et al. A multicenter randomized controlled trial of Zephyr Endobronchial valve treatment in heterogeneous emphysema (LIBERATE). Am J Respir Crit Care Med. 2018;198(9):1151–64.
5. Kemp SV, Slebos DJ, Kirk A, Kornaszewska M, Carron K, Ek L, et al. A multicenter randomized controlled trial of Zephyr Endobronchial valve treatment in heterogeneous emphysema (TRANSFORM). Am J Respir Crit Care Med. 2017;196(12):1535–43.
6. Magnussen H, Kramer MR, Kirsten AM, Marquette C, Valipour A, Stanzel F, et al. Effect of fissure integrity on lung volume reduction using a polymer sealant in advanced emphysema. Thorax. 2012;67(4):302–8.
7. Criner GJ, Delage A, Voelker K, Hogarth DK, Majid A, Zgoda M, et al. Improving lung function in severe heterogenous emphysema with the spiration valve system (EMPROVE). A multicenter, open-label randomized controlled clinical trial. Am J Respir Crit Care Med. 2019;200(11):1354–62.

8. Deslee G, Mal H, Dutau H, Bourdin A, Vergnon JM, Pison C, et al. Lung volume reduction coil treatment vs usual Care in Patients with Severe Emphysema: the REVOLENS randomized clinical trial. JAMA. 2016;315(2):175–84.
9. Abia-Trujillo D, Yu Lee-Mateus A, Garcia-Saucedo JC, Saifi O, Patel NM, Herth FJF, et al. Prevention of acute exacerbation of chronic obstructive pulmonary disease after bronchoscopic lung volume reduction with endobronchial valves. Clin Respir J. 2022;16(1):43–8.
10. Fiorelli A, D'Andrilli A, Bezzi M, Ibrahim M, Anile M, Diso D, et al. Complications related to endoscopic lung volume reduction for emphysema with endobronchial valves: results of a multicenter study. J Thorac Dis. 2018;10(Suppl 27):S3315–S25.
11. Lee EG, Rhee CK. Bronchoscopic lung volume reduction using an endobronchial valve to treat a huge emphysematous bullae: a case report. BMC Pulm Med. 2019;19(1):92.
12. Elayaperumal AK, Jackson RE. Anaesthesia for lung volume reduction surgery and endobronchial valves. BJA Educ. 2018;18(7):193–8.
13. Koster TD, Slebos DJ. The fissure: interlobar collateral ventilation and implications for endoscopic therapy in emphysema. Int J Chron Obstruct Pulmon Dis. 2016;11:765–73.

Anesthesia for Patients with Hemoptysis/Massive Hemoptysis

11

Anastasia Katsiampoura

11.1 Introduction

Physicians have long acknowledged massive hemoptysis as an urgent and challenging condition. It was in the late 1940s that surgical interventions with potential clinical benefits were first documented [1]. Due to the critical nature of massive hemoptysis, the treatment approach was aggressive, often necessitating urgent surgical intervention via thoracotomy once the bleeding site was localized. However, advancements in interventional pulmonology (IP) and interventional radiology have transformed the treatment algorithm for massive hemoptysis. The field of interventional pulmonology has advanced over the last couple of decades with new technology.

Massive hemoptysis is the life-threatening expectoration of large volumes of blood as a result of a tumor, infection, or other cause. Historically, it has been managed with emergent thoracotomy. Endobronchial and endovascular therapies are now often utilized as temporizing measures to control bleeding and bridge to more definitive therapies such as chemotherapy, antibiotics, or surgery. Depending on the underlying pathology's anatomical location, the case's complexity, the operator's expertise and preference, and local availability, these can be applied with flexible or rigid bronchoscopy or a combination of both. Management can be complex and is best handled by a well-trained, multidisciplinary team with specialized anesthetic support.

This chapter reviews a detailed, modern approach to managing massive hemoptysis in the interventional pulmonology suite.

A. Katsiampoura (✉)
Department of Anesthesia, Critical Care and Pain Medicine, Beth Israel Deaconess Medical Center, Harvard Medical School, Boston, MA, USA
e-mail: akatsiam@bidmc.harvard.edu

M. Sarkiss (ed.), *Anesthesia for Interventional Pulmonary Procedures*,
https://doi.org/10.1007/978-3-032-12007-6_11

11.2 Definitions of Hemoptysis and Massive Hemoptysis

Hemoptysis, the coughing up blood from the respiratory tract, is a common reason for hospital consultation [2]. Hemoptysis can be classified into different levels, ranging from mild, with slight traces of blood in the sputum, to moderate, with more significant amounts of blood and possible mild changes in blood circulation [3]. On the other hand, massive hemoptysis, which involves the expectoration of over 300 ml of blood in a day, presents a life-threatening situation, leading to severe breathing difficulties and unstable blood circulation [2–4]. It is imperative to discern hemoptysis from other forms of bleeding, such as hematemesis originating from the gastrointestinal tract. The severity of hemoptysis guides its categorization, with life-threatening hemoptysis causing significant respiratory impairment and jeopardizing life.

11.3 Pulmonary Vascular Anatomy

The lungs are supplied by two different vascular circulations: the pulmonary and the bronchial systems. The primary function of the pulmonary system is to oxygenate blood by exchanging gases between the lungs and the blood, a process that also involves removeing carbon dioxide fromthe body. The literature defines severe or massive hemoptysis based on the amount of blood expected to be produced within 24 hours [5]. However, there has yet to be an agreement on a specific threshold for classifying hemoptysis as massive. Different studies use different thresholds, ranging from 100 mL to over 1000 mL [6]. These definitions could be better due to the challenges associated with reported volumes, which may be overestimated or underestimated. Unfortunately, obtaining such precise measurements is usually not feasible during the initial presentation [7]. Another definition of Massive hemoptysis focuses on the magnitude of the effect of the volume of expectorated blood that is life-threatening due to airway obstruction, hypotension, or blood loss [8–10]. This definition relies on the main clinical consequence of hemoptysis; examples of such a definition have included hemoptysis requiring transfusion, hospitalization, intubation, aspiration of blood to the contralateral lung, airway obstruction, hypoxemia requiring mechanical ventilation ($PaO2 < 60$ mmHg), and death [1, 2].

The incidence of massive hemoptysis is less than 20%, with various causes contributing to this severe complication. Although it accounts for 10–15% of hemoptysis episodes, if the bleeding is not controlled, it has a mortality rate of over 50%.

Morbidity and mortality in hemoptysis patients depend on the volume of expectorated blood, the rate of bleeding, the timeliness of hemoptysis management, and the extent and severity of any underlying disease reducing one's cardiopulmonary reserve. Hypoxemia is the primary cause of heightened mortality in patients who exhibit hemoptysis. This is considered more dangerous than exsanguination or blood loss through bleeding.

Despite thorough investigations, a significant proportion of hemoptysis remains cryptogenic, emphasizing the need for continuous research and improved diagnostic strategies.

The broncial arteries supplu blood to the tracheobronchial tree and other structures down to the terminal bronchioles. These arteries branch from the thoracic aorta and deliver oxygenated blood for the nutritional needs of the airways, while the pulmonary arteries are responsibel for gas exchange. These two systems also flow blood to hilar lymph nodes, visceral pleura, pulmonary arteries and veins, vagus nerve, and esophagus [11].

The pulmonary arterial system operates at low pressure (with normal systolic pressures of 15–20 mmHg and diastolic pressures of 5–10 mmHg), carrying blood from the right ventricle across the pulmonary capillary bed and returning it via the pulmonary veins to the left atrium. The pulmonary arteries only interact with the airway at the level of the terminal bronchioles, where they bronch extensively around the alveoli to facilitate efficient gas exchange [12].

The pulmonary arteries contribute 99% of the blood supply to the lungs, while the bronchial arteries provide the remaining 1%. An anastomosis between these arteries can result in right-to-left shunts. Reduction in pulmonary blood supply can prompt an increased supply from bronchial arteries, particularly in conditions such as thromboembolism and inflammation. Common causes of hemoptysis include bronchiectasis, chronic bronchitis, tuberculosis, and malignancy [3, 13, 14].

The increased vascularization of lung parenchyma by bronchial and nonbronchial systemic arteries underlies the cause of hemoptysis. Common culprits for hemoptysis include infections (such as tuberculosis or fungal infections), chronic bronchitis, bronchiectasis, and malignancy.

The vascular sources of hemoptysis are categorized into bronchial (90%) and nonbronchial (10%). Bronchial arteries are the primary instigators in over 90% of cases [15]. In addition to pulmonary causes, nonpulmonary contributors to hemoptysis encompass numerous conditions. For instance, cardiac abnormalities like left ventricular failure and mitral stenosis, gastrointestinal disorders like gastroesophageal reflux disease, and systemic conditions including coagulopathies and autoimmune disorders can all lead to hemoptysis [16, 17]. Addressing the underlying conditions contributing to hemoptysis is crucial for a holistic therapeutic approach.

11.4 Bronchial Causes of Hemoptysis

Various pulmonary conditions, such as bronchiectasis, lung cancer, tuberculosis, and mycetomas, have different prevalence rates across different centers. These conditions can also be iatrogenic after a biopsy. It may occur due to traumatic events such as chest trauma, postsurgical complications, or idiopathic factors. The pulmonary artery may also be implicated in hemoptysis due to infection, trauma, or vasculitis [17]. Inflammatory disorders like vasculitis and granulomatosis with polyangiitis can also trigger hemoptysis.

Some less common causes of hemoptysis include left ventricular aneurysms, which are often associated with myocardial infarction, cardiac surgery, or infection [18]. A rare developmental anomaly known as proximal interruption of the pulmonary artery can be addressed through pneumonectomy or anastomosis [19, 20].

Hemoptysis as a bronchoscopy complication is rare but can range from 0.26% to 5%, influenced by patient risk factors such as malignancy, coagulopathy, and immunocompromised states [21].

11.5 Nonbronchial Causes of Hemoptysis

Nonbronchial systemic arteries contributing to hemoptysis include the brachiocephalic artery, subclavian artery, thyrocervical trunk, costocervical artery, axillary artery, intercostal arteries, inferior phrenic artery, gastric artery, and branches of the celiac axis [17]. These sources can be effectively managed with transcatheter embolization. Pseudoaneurysms of the internal mammary artery and costocervical artery, causing hemoptysis, are also successfully treated with endovascular embolization. Other nonbronchial causes involve pulmonary artery pathologies such as pulmonary emboli, Rasmussen's aneurysm, Dieulafoy's disease, and pulmonary arteriovenous malformations (AVMs).

11.6 Clinical Presentation and Severity Assessment

The manifestation of hemoptysis in clinical presentation often includes symptoms such as coughing up blood, chest pain, shortness of breath, weakness, or fatigue. Assessing the severity of hemoptysis involves evaluating multiple factors, including the volume of expectorated blood (categorized as mild, moderate, or massive), the patient's hemodynamic stability, respiratory distress or compromise, and any underlying conditions exacerbating the situation [22].

The severity assessment encompasses evaluating the volume of expectorated blood, determining hemodynamic stability, identifying signs indicating respiratory distress or compromise, and considering underlying health conditions. Diagnostic tools provide additional insights, including imaging studies such as chest X-ray, CT scan, bronchoscopy, and laboratory tests like CBC, coagulation profile, and ABG analysis. A comprehensive clinical history and physical examination are essential to explore risk factors, smoking history, recent infections, and preexisting pulmonary or systemic conditions [23].

11.7 Management of Hemoptysis in the IP Suite

Patients can present with hemoptysis in the interventional pulmonology suite as their primary diagnosis or as the result of an intervention. The IP suite is an exclusive realm for hemoptysis. The performance of transbronchial biopsies is linked to an escalated vulnerability to iatrogenic hemoptysis.

Rapid and simultaneous diagnostic and therapeutic interventions are necessary to manage massive hemoptysis. In cases where a patient is coughing up a significant amount of blood but can still prevent it from entering their lungs and maintaining normal oxygen saturation levels without any respiratory distress, they are considered stable. Despite the often-frightening appearance, these patients are defending their lungs. This is usually not pertinent when patients have already received anesthesia for a procedure in the IP suite. The primary concern is the patient's respiratory condition, including their respiratory rate, oxygen saturation levels, and potential for respiratory distress, rather than their hemoglobin levels [24].

Endovascular management, specifically embolization of bronchial arteries, is usually the first-line treatment to control the bleeding. Hemoptysis may require endovascular treatment if its volume exceeds 200 mL in 24–48 hours, causes acute respiratory failure, or if the mechanism is potentially life-threatening, such as pulmonary artery erosion [2].

Parallel, bronchoscopy is an essential intervention in managing life-threatening hemoptysis. It can be used for diagnostic and therapeutic purposes and performed quickly at the bedside. It is readily available after an intervention in the IP suite [1].

11.7.1 Pseudo-hemoptysis

It is defined as the expectoration of blood originating from the nasopharynx, oropharynx, larynx, or gastrointestinal tract. This must be recognized because an entirely different diagnostic algorithm is required [25].

11.7.2 Preoperative Assessment and Diagnostic Workup

A comprehensive preoperative assessment is essential for thoroughly evaluating the patient's health status and potential risk factors (Fig. 11.1). This assessment involves careful risk stratification and evaluation of any existing medical conditions that could affect the time around the surgery. The choice between general and regional anesthesia depends on the patient's condition and the type of surgery being performed.

Before the procedure for a patient who presents with bleeding, it is essential to identify the urgency of the procedure. Gathering a detailed history to determine the cause and source of bleeding is necessary if time allows. It is crucial first to confirm whether the lower respiratory tract is the source of bleeding as nonrespiratory causes rarely lead to hemoptysis. Specific questions and physical exams are necessary to rule out upper respiratory or gastrointestinal bleeding. Quantifying the amount and rate of bleeding is essential as it determines the urgency and scope of further testing. The history should also include details about the sputum, any related pulmonary symptoms, and relevant medical history, such as prior pulmonary conditions, trauma, and exposure to harmful substances. Additionally, the patient's age can offer valuable insights as certain conditions are more common in specific age groups.

The selection of diagnostic tests for investigating and locating the source of hemoptysis depends on the patient's medical history and current clinical presentation. Performing a complete blood count (CBC), arterial blood gas analysis (ABG),

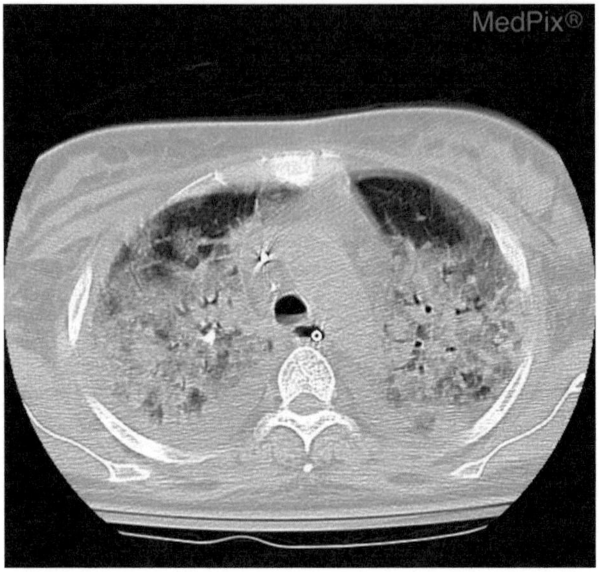

Fig. 11.1 CT scan of a patient with intrapulmonary hemorrhage. (https://openi.nlm.nih.gov/detailedresult?img=MPX2115_synpic21666&query=&req=4)

and coagulation profile is recommended. In cases where diffuse alveolar hemorrhage is suspected, urinalysis, ESR, and CRP tests can help identify hemoptysis's underlying cause and severity [26].

In hemoptysis, pinpointing the exact cause can be challenging due to potential blood movement. Thus, consider performing a STAT chest X-ray even if a chest CT has already been requested (Fig. 11.2). Research has shown that a chest X-ray can help locate the bleeding site in around 46% of cases and identify the specific cause in approximately 35% of cases [3]. However, further exploration is often necessary, particularly when there are known risk factors for lung cancer and a routine chest X-ray [3] (Fig. 11.3).

11.7.3 Intraoperative

Coordination among the anesthesia team, interventional pulmonologists, and healthcare providers is crucial for effective communication and swift responses to unforeseen events, such as massive bleeding or respiratory compromise in the interventional pulmonology suite.

Being familiar with the procedural layout is also crucial, especially in hospitals where interventional pulmonary (IP) rooms may be outside the main operating rooms, posing limited access and assistance challenges.

When a patient experiences hemoptysis, immediate therapeutic interventions are crucial. These interventions include preserving respiratory function and

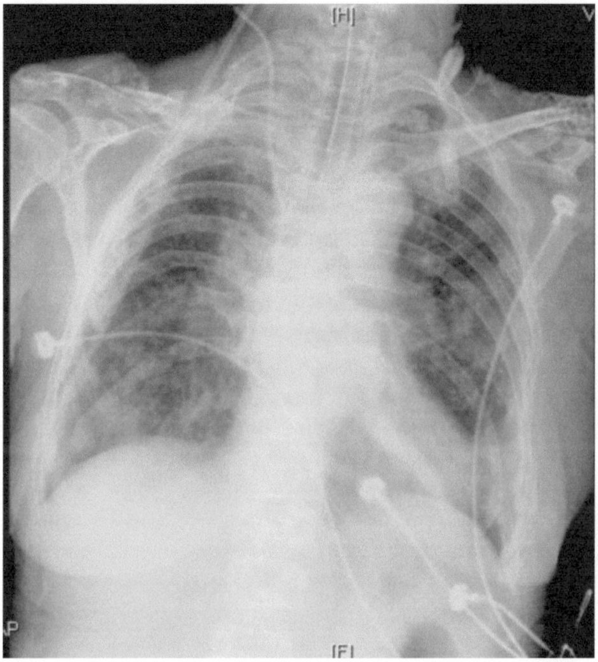

Fig. 11.2 X-ray of a patient with massive hemoptysis. (https://openi.nlm.nih.gov/detailedresult?img=MPX2115_synpic21666&query=&req=4, https://creativecommons.org/licenses/by/2.0/)

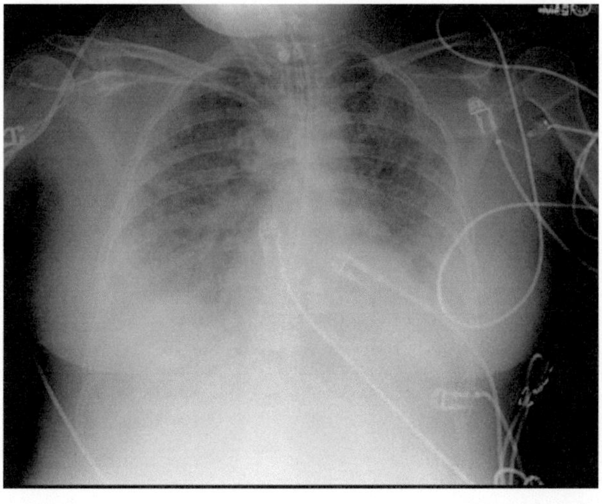

Fig. 11.3 X-ray of a patient with massive hemoptysis. (https://openi.nlm.nih.gov/detailedresult?img=PMC2772246_IJCCM-13-96-g001&query=intrapulmonary%20hemorrhage&it=xg&req=4&npos=23)

preventing blood from entering the lungs by using an endobronchial blocker and positioning the patient on the nonbleeding side. Stopping the bleeding at its source can be achieved through coagulation manipulation or direct intervention. Diagnosing the underlying cause and planning the next steps are also important considerations. It is essential to note that these interventions should co-occur without a specific order.

Continuous monitoring of the patient's vital signs, including blood pressure, heart rate, oxygen saturation, and temperature, is essential during anesthesia. Capnography is recommended for monitoring the patient's breathing. However, this is only sometimes feasible in the IP suite. ETCO2 monitoring is usually unreliable during bronchoscopy, and there is frequent endobronchial suctioning.

Vigilance during bronchoscopy is crucial to anticipate acute bleeding risks. Awareness of the specific bronchoscopy location enables timely intervention (Fig. 11.4).

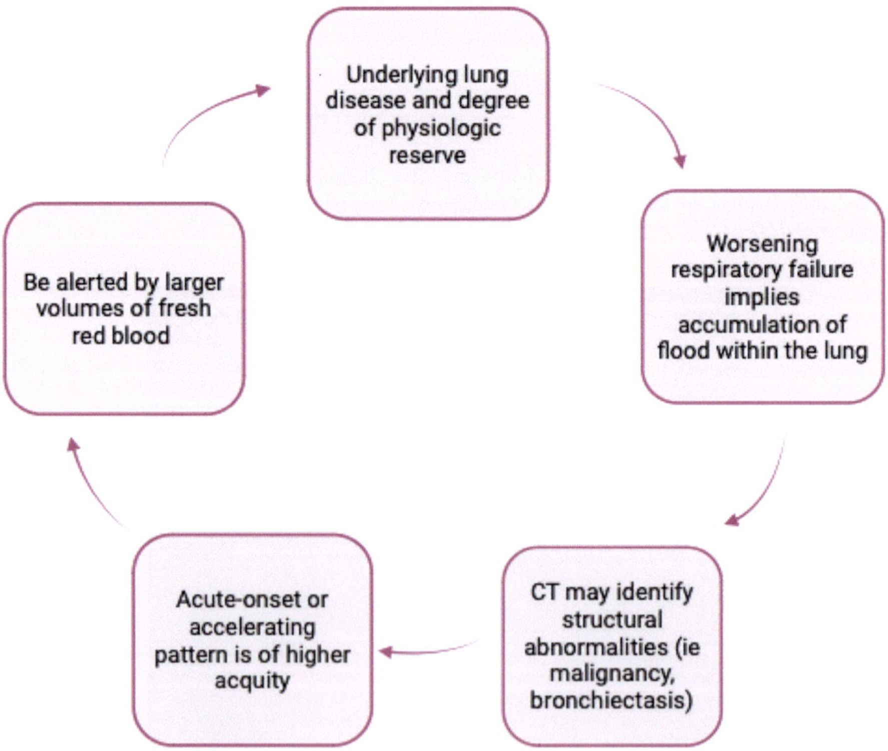

Fig. 11.4 Hints for clinical assessment of a patient with intrapulmonary hemorrhage. (Figure illustration T. Constantinou)

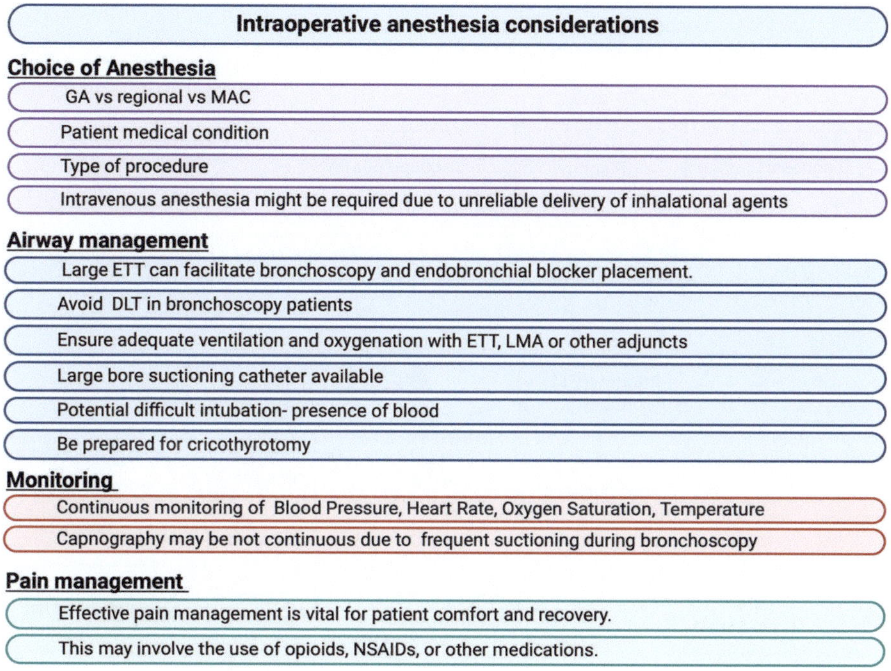

Fig. 11.5 Intraoperative anesthesia considerations. (Figure illustration T. Constantinou)

11.7.4 Anesthesia Management

Critical considerations for anesthesia management include IV access, central line insertion, lung isolation techniques, and arterial line placement.

The choice of anesthesia depends on factors such as the patient's medical condition, the type of intervention, and the proceduralist's preference. Proper airway management is essential for ensuring adequate ventilation and oxygenation during surgery. This may involve using an endotracheal tube, laryngeal mask airway, or other adjuncts. Options include general anesthesia, regional anesthesia, and monitored anesthesia care. GA is recommended in most cases with intrapulmonary hemorrhage (Fig. 11.5).

11.7.5 Indications for Intubation

Intubation may be necessary in cases of respiratory failure. Signs of an ineffective cough include gurgling and an inability to clear blood from the airway. Worsening respiratory failure may manifest as hypoxemia and dyspnea. Intubation can be required for respiratory failure or to expedite the IP procedure (Fig. 11.6). The induction of GA should consider the hemodynamic conditions and fast-optimize the conditions for intubation. Considerations should include the risk of aspiration in

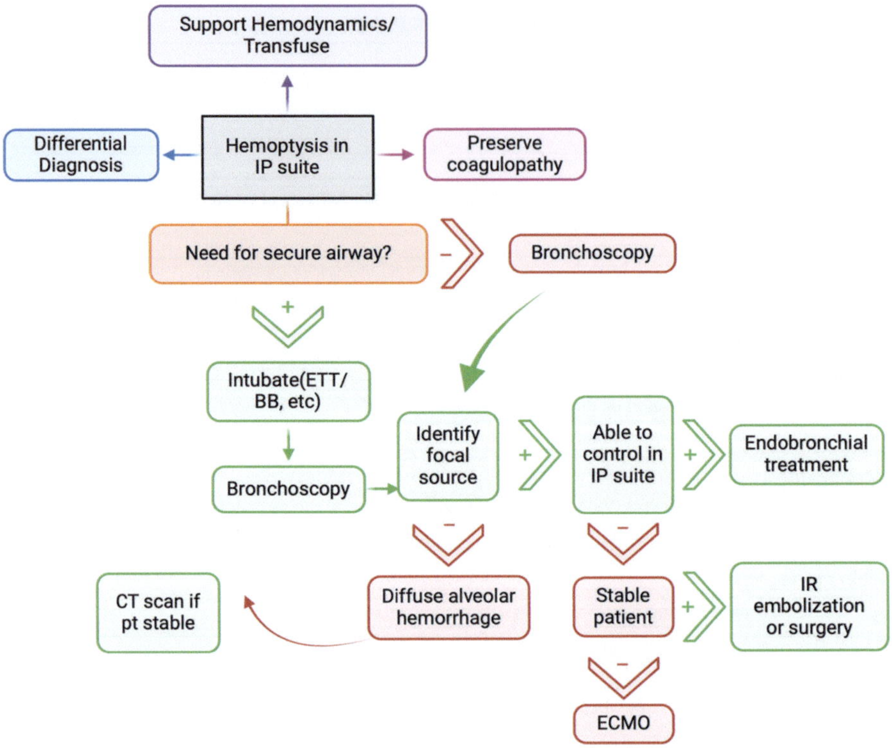

Fig. 11.6 Intraoperative management algorithm for hemoptysis in the IP suite. (Figure illustration T. Constantinou)

situations such as when the patient has been swallowing blood. In this case, rapid sequence induction (RSI) is indicated. Due to the unreliable delivery of the inhalational agents, maintenance of anesthesia should be accomplished with total intravenous anesthetic (TIVA).

11.7.6 Nonintubated Bronchoscopy ("Awake Branch")

Nonintubated bronchoscopy may be selected when the patient can preserve their cough reflex, enabling them to clear blood from their lungs after the procedure. The primary objective is to identify a specific source of bleeding, if it exists, or to assess whether the patient may be experiencing diffuse alveolar hemorrhage [27].

11.7.7 Intubated Bronchoscopy

In certain situations, prioritizing airway patency and endotracheal intubation may be required before a procedure or rigid bronchoscopy. If endotracheal intubation is chosen, profound sedation, such as a high-dose propofol infusion, can make it easier to access the area because the patient will not cough and move blood around. A stable lung will also make determining the source of bleeding easier [28, 29].

It is crucial to secure the airway early, especially in cases with a risk of aspiration, such as when a patient has been swallowing blood. Quick identification and response to compromised airways due to bleeding or underlying pathology is essential. It is also important to have contingency plans to promptly identify and manage intraoperative and postoperative complications related to hemoptysis.

When preparing for intubation, it is important to anticipate potential difficulties due to blood, making it challenging to locate anatomical landmarks. It is advisable to have a large-bore suction catheter ready for suctioning and be prepared for cricothyrotomy if the airway becomes obstructed by blood and landmarks are not visible. For intubation, using an oversized endotracheal tube (ETT) is recommended. For average-sized or taller patients, it is suggested to use a #9 ETT, and alternatively, an 8.5 mm ETT or more significant can be used. It is essential to use a sizeable endotracheal tube to facilitate the passage of a therapeutic flexible bronchoscope, which is preferred in hemoptysis cases due to its more significant working channel, providing superior suction capabilities [30].

Selective endobronchial intubation (SEI) is a more straightforward and cost-effective technique, but it carries the risk of tube migration, especially in the right mainstem bronchus.

Bronchial blockers like Cohen, Arndt, and Univent offer the advantage of isolating specific lobes or segments but require deflation for distal exploration.

"Balloon tamponade may help stop bleeding if the bleeding is confined to a specific lung, lobe, or segment. The aim is to categorize the bleeding and safeguard the rest of the lung tissue. Either paralysis or deep sedation (such as a propofol infusion) is typically required to prevent the patient from coughing or dislodging the tamponade."

Double lumen tubes (DLTs), which have two lumens, allow for the ventilation of both lungs but require technical expertise in proper positioning [31].

11.8 Treatment Modalities for Managing Intrapulmonary Hemorrhage

Dealing with hemoptysis necessitates a holistic strategy incorporating medical, interventional, and surgical techniques (Fig. 11.7). Medical interventions focus on halting bleeding, while minimally invasive interventional radiology methods, such as embolization, aim to block blood flow to the affected area. Surgical interventions, such as lobectomy, wedge resection, or other procedures, may be essential for cases requiring more conclusive treatment.

Traditional treatment options for massive hemoptysis included lobectomy or pneumonectomy and bronchial artery ligation. However, these procedures carried high risks. Over the years, less invasive interventional pulmonary procedures have been developed, such as endobronchial therapies and advanced imaging and navigation techniques (e.g., the ION robot). These advancements have significantly improved patient outcomes by reducing the need for high-risk surgeries.

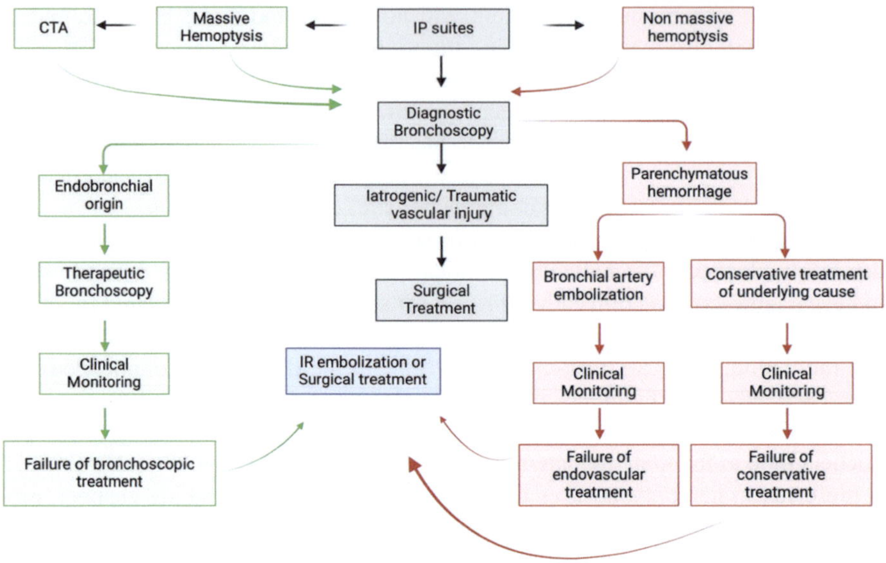

Fig. 11.7 Treatment modalities for the management of hemoptysis. (Figure illustration T. Constantinou)

11.8.1 Bronchoscopy

It is important to remember that bronchoscopy is a crucial procedure for diagnosing and treating hemoptysis. A skilled bronchoscopic team and proper equipment are essential for ensuring the safe performance of bronchoscopy, especially in cases of severe hemoptysis [32].

One critical benefit of bronchoscopy is its ability to identify the specific source of bleeding, such as an endobronchial tumor or blood from a single airway. However, this can be challenging [2]. While CT scans are increasingly being utilized as the primary method to locate bleeding due to their accuracy compared to bronchoscopy, the availability of bronchoscopy is valuable for patients with intrapulmonary hemorrhage in the IP suite [33, 34].

Additionally, bronchoscopy can assist in diagnosing diffuse alveolar hemorrhage, characterized by bleeding from all airways that do not clear with sequential lavage. In some cases, it is also used to deploy an endobronchial blocker to control bleeding [35]. Performing bronchoscopy on intubated patients with hemoptysis is recommended to evaluate the severity of bleeding and apply tamponade if necessary. Furthermore, it may be conducted when the source of bleeding remains unclear despite CT scan findings.

The bronchoscopist may need to address iatrogenic bleeding resulting from procedures like transbronchial biopsies, where significant bleeding occurs in approximately 2.8% of cases [36]. For non-iatrogenic hemoptysis cases, flexible bronchoscopy becomes an indispensable procedure, enabling the identification of the bleeding source, endoscopic treatment, and the ability to perform pulmonary isolation to safeguard the unaffected lung.

Rigid bronchoscopy allows bronchoscopists to perform local tamponade for centrally located bleeding sources and employ various endoscopic techniques. It also permits selective intubation for pulmonary isolation in cases of catastrophic bleeding [37].

The conventional method for managing endobronchial bleeding involved using cold saline, epinephrine, or activated factor VIIa. However, activated factor VIIa is costly, while epinephrine, although somewhat effective, is also systemically absorbed, and cold saline needs to be deemed adequate. In recent years, various bronchoscopic techniques have demonstrated promising success rates in treating significant hemorrhages. Endobronchial tranexamic acid is considered a potentially better alternative, although there is limited evidence to substantiate this [38]. Several other diagnostic bronchoscopy interventions have been studied for controlling hemoptysis during interventional pulmonary procedures. These methods include cold saline lavage, vasopressin analogs, oxidized regenerated cellulose (ORC) mesh, and glue treatment. Cold saline lavage has been used to control bleeding, although large-volume cold saline lavages have yet to be widely studied in recent trials [37].

ORC mesh has been used as a topical hemostatic agent, achieving immediate hemorrhage control in most patients. However, absorption and postobstructive pneumonia were observed in some cases. Glue treatment also achieved immediate control of hemoptysis with no recurrences observed in a 6-month follow-up study [39]. Vasopressin analogs effectively control hemoptysis, with intravenous administration resulting in a significantly higher diastolic pressure than endobronchial administration. These methods offer potential options for managing hemoptysis, and medical research is ongoing.

11.8.2 Endobronchial Stents

Endobronchial stents have proven effective in treating hemoptysis caused by endobronchial lesions, common in advanced lung cancer. These stents are used as a palliative measure. Reports indicate that both silicone and covered self-expandable metal stents have positive immediate outcomes [40].

Endobronchial embolization using silicone spigots (EESS) is a procedure used to control bleeding in segmental airways. It was introduced by Dutau et al. [41] The process involves identifying the bleeding segment and utilizing biopsy forceps to insert a fixture through the working channel of a flexible bronchoscope. Sometimes, airway stabilization with a rigid bronchoscope is performed before flexible bronchoscopy. The fixture is then placed to block the bleeding segmental airway. Several case reports have described EESS being used in various medical conditions [37]. Kho et al. presented a study on the use of EESS in the treatment of hemoptysis [42].

11.8.3 Laser Photocoagulation

In 1982, Dumon et al. introduced laser photocoagulation, significantly changing bronchoscopic procedures. Medical lasers are now widely available and differ mainly in their wavelength, determining their effect on treated tissue. Nd: YAG and Nd:YAP lasers are commonly used in bronchoscopy due to their superior coagulation effects, while CO2 lasers, with a significantly higher wavelength of 10,600 nm, are more suitable for cutting impacts [43].

Han et al. conducted a retrospective review to assess the effectiveness of laser treatment in patients with central airway tumors. The study revealed promising results, with laser treatment achieving complete resolution in 77% of patients with hemoptysis. In addition, partial improvement was observed in 17% of patients, and no procedure-related mortality was reported among 110 patients [44]. Another study focusing on endoscopic palliative treatment for tracheobronchial tumors showed a relatively lower short-term efficacy rate, with 58% of patients being free of hemoptysis for at least 1 month after laser treatment. Case reports also highlight the effectiveness of lasers in addressing significant hemoptysis resulting from large central lesions [45].

11.8.4 Argon Plasma Coagulation

Argon plasma is a method used in the medical field that employs ionized gas atoms to carry electrical currents in lesions found in the airways. This method transforms electrical current into thermal energy upon contact with a tumor, leading to its coagulation. Argon plasma coagulation surpasses laser photocoagulation as it can address lesions regardless of their orientation to the probe. A retrospective review by Morice et al. indicated that argon plasma achieved a 100% immediate bleeding control rate in patients with endobronchial lesions and hemoptysis, and there were no recurrences over an average follow-up period of 97 ± 92 days. Besides its use in treating endobronchial tumors, argon plasma coagulation effectively addresses hemangiomas and endobronchial endometriosis [46].

11.8.5 Tranexamic Acid

Tranexamic acid (TXA) is a medication that hinders the breakdown of blood clots and has demonstrated potential in reducing the duration and amount of bleeding in cases of hemoptysis. Although studies have varied in their designs and the groups they focused on, TXA is linked to shortened bleeding duration, as proven in controlled trials [47]. TXA can be administered through different means, such as orally and intravenously. Moreover, novel methods like aerosolization and endobronchial instillation have shown promising results. However, it is essential to note that while TXA is a viable option to manage bleeding while waiting for other treatments or tests, it should not be regarded as the definitive therapy and should not delay or obstruct other interventions. It is more suitable for patients on the relatively stable end of the hemoptysis spectrum. A reasonable dose of nebulized TXA could be 500 mg every 8 hours, with an initial dose of 1000 mg. Furthermore, TXA seems safe and well-tolerated, but further well-designed clinical studies are needed to understand its effectiveness and safety profile comprehensively [48].

11.8.6 Endobronchial Valves

The endobronchial valves were first created for endoscopic lung volume reduction in patients with emphysema [49]. They offer a new treatment method, allowing air to exit a pulmonary lobe while preventing air from entering, which can lead to atelectasis if collateral ventilation is lacking. While these valves are mainly used for reducing lung volume, there are two documented cases where they were effectively used to address severe hemoptysis in patients with tuberculosis complications [50]. However, caution is necessary when using these valves due to the risk of pneumothorax after valve placement, which can present significant difficulties in severe hemoptysis cases [37].

11.8.7 DDAVP, Fibrinogen, and Coagulation

In cases of hemoptysis, it is essential to manage hypofibrinogenemia by administering cryoprecipitate or fibrinogen concentrate to achieve a fibrinogen level greater than 150 mg/dL. In cases where patients are on antiplatelet agents or have renal failure leading to platelet dysfunction, desmopressin (DDAVP) at a dose of 0.3 ug/kg may be considered [51]. Additionally, any anticoagulants should be reversed whenever possible. To address thrombocytopenia, it is recommended that platelet transfusion be administered to achieve a platelet count greater than 50,000 per microliter [52].

References

1. Radchenko C, Alraiyes AH, Shojaee S. A systematic approach to the management of massive hemoptysis. J Thorac Dis. 2017;9(Suppl 10):S1069–S86.
2. Sakr L, Dutau H. Massive hemoptysis: an update on the role of bronchoscopy in diagnosis and management. Respiration. 2010;80(1):38–58.
3. Larici AR, Franchi P, Occhipinti M, Contegiacomo A, del Ciello A, Calandriello L, et al. Diagnosis and management of hemoptysis. Diagn Interv Radiol. 2014;20(4):299–309.
4. Britto MT, Kotagal UR, Hornung RW, Atherton HD, Tsevat J, Wilmott RW. Impact of recent pulmonary exacerbations on quality of life in patients with cystic fibrosis. Chest. 2002;121(1):64–72.
5. Hirshberg B, Biran I, Glazer M, Kramer MR. Hemoptysis: etiology, evaluation, and outcome in a tertiary referral hospital. Chest. 1997;112(2):440–4.
6. Cordovilla R, Bollo de Miguel E, Nunez Ares A, Cosano Povedano FJ, Herraez Ortega I, Jimenez MR. Diagnosis and treatment of hemoptysis. Arch Bronconeumol. 2016;52(7):368–77.

7. Dudha M, Lehrman S, Aronow WS, Rosa J. Hemoptysis: diagnosis and treatment. Compr Ther. 2009;35(3–4):139–49.
8. Garzon AA, Cerruti MM, Golding ME. Exsanguinating hemoptysis. J Thorac Cardiovasc Surg. 1982;84(6):829–33.
9. Flume PA, Yankaskas JR, Ebeling M, Hulsey T, Clark LL. Massive hemoptysis in cystic fibrosis. Chest. 2005;128(2):729–38.
10. Ibrahim WH. Massive haemoptysis: the definition should be revised. Eur Respir J. 2008;32(4):1131–2.
11. Chaudhry R, Omole AE, Bordoni B. Anatomy, thorax, lungs. Treasure Island (FL): StatPearls; 2025.
12. Kandathil A, Chamarthy M. Pulmonary vascular anatomy & anatomical variants. Cardiovasc Diagn Ther. 2018;8(3):201–7.
13. Gupta A, Sands M, Chauhan NR. Massive hemoptysis in pulmonary infections: bronchial artery embolization. J Thorac Dis. 2018;10(Suppl 28):S3458–s64.
14. Almeida J, Leal C, Figueiredo L. Evaluation of the bronchial arteries: normal findings, hypertrophy and embolization in patients with hemoptysis. Insights Imaging. 2020;11(1):70.
15. Swanson KL, Johnson CM, Prakash UB, McKusick MA, Andrews JC, Stanson AW. Bronchial artery embolization : experience with 54 patients. Chest. 2002;121(3):789–95.
16. Salama AD, Levy JB, Lightstone L, Pusey CD. Goodpasture's disease. Lancet. 2001;358(9285):917–20.
17. Singhal M, Lal A, Prabhakar N, Yadav MK, Vijayvergiya R, Behra D, et al. Non-bronchial causes of haemoptysis: imaging and interventions. Pol J Radiol. 2020;85:e328–e39.
18. Corr P. Pulmonary artery aneurysm as a cause of massive hemoptysis: diagnosis and management. Case Rep Radiol. 2011;2011:141563.
19. Mattioni G, Nosotti M, Rosso L, Palleschi A, Tosi D, Mendogni P. Pneumonectomy for unilateral proximal interruption of pulmonary artery: a case series from the literature. Life (Basel). 2023;13(12).
20. Anand SH, Jasper A, Mani SE, Joseph E, Mathai J. Proximal interruption of the pulmonary artery: a case series. J Clin Diagn Res. 2015;9(12):TD04–6.
21. Tai R, Dunne RM, Trotman-Dickenson B, Jacobson FL, Madan R, Kumamaru KK, et al. Frequency and severity of pulmonary hemorrhage in patients undergoing percutaneous CT-guided transthoracic lung biopsy: single-institution experience of 1175 cases. Radiology. 2016;279(1):287–96.
22. O'Gurek D, Choi HYJ. Hemoptysis: evaluation and management. Am Fam Physician. 2022;105(2):144–51.
23. Sevransky J. Clinical assessment of hemodynamically unstable patients. Curr Opin Crit Care. 2009;15(3):234–8.
24. Kathuria H, Hollingsworth HM, Vilvendhan R, Reardon C. Management of life-threatening hemoptysis. J Intensive Care. 2020;8:23.
25. DiLeo MD, Amedee RG, Butcher RB. Hemoptysis and pseudohemoptysis: the patient expectorating blood. Ear Nose Throat J. 1995;74(12):822–4, 6, 8, passim.
26. Ittrich H, Bockhorn M, Klose H, Simon M. The diagnosis and treatment of hemoptysis. Dtsch Arztebl Int. 2017;114(21):371–81.
27. Patolia S, Farhat R, Subramaniyam R. Bronchoscopy in intubated and non-intubated intensive care unit patients with respiratory failure. J Thorac Dis. 2021;13(8):5125–34.
28. Galway U, Zura A, Khanna S, Wang M, Turan A, Ruetzler K. Anesthetic considerations for bronchoscopic procedures: a narrative review based on the Cleveland Clinic experience. J Thorac Dis. 2019;11(7):3156–70.
29. José RJ, Shaefi S, Navani N. Anesthesia for bronchoscopy. Curr Opin Anaesthesiol. 2014;27(4):453–7.
30. Law JA, Broemling N, Cooper RM, Drolet P, Duggan LV, Griesdale DE, et al. The difficult airway with recommendations for management--part 1--difficult tracheal intubation encountered in an unconscious/induced patient. Can J Anaesth. 2013;60(11):1089–118.

31. Correia S, Dionísio J, Duro da Costa JJ. Modified technique of endobronchial balloon tamponade for persistent hemoptysis. J Bronchol Interv Pulmonol. 2014;21(4):361–5.
32. Mohan A, Madan K, Hadda V, Tiwari P, Mittal S, Guleria R, et al. Guidelines for diagnostic flexible bronchoscopy in adults: joint Indian Chest Society/National College of chest physicians (I)/Indian association for bronchology recommendations. Lung India. 2019;36(Supplement):S37–89.
33. Revel MP, Fournier LS, Hennebicque AS, Cuenod CA, Meyer G, Reynaud P, et al. Can CT replace bronchoscopy in the detection of the site and cause of bleeding in patients with large or massive hemoptysis? AJR Am J Roentgenol. 2002;179(5):1217–24.
34. Mondoni M, Carlucci P, Cipolla G, Fois A, Gasparini S, Marani S, et al. Bronchoscopy to assess patients with hemoptysis: which is the optimal timing? BMC Pulm Med. 2019;19(1):36.
35. Park MS. Diffuse alveolar hemorrhage. Tuberc Respir Dis (Seoul). 2013;74(4):151–62.
36. Bernasconi M, Koegelenberg CFN, Koutsokera A, Ogna A, Casutt A, Nicod L, et al. Iatrogenic bleeding during flexible bronchoscopy: risk factors, prophylactic measures and management. ERJ Open Res. 2017;3(2):00084.
37. Gagnon S, Quigley N, Dutau H, Delage A, Fortin M. Approach to hemoptysis in the modern era. Can Respir J. 2017;2017:1565030.
38. Moen CA, Burrell A, Dunning J. Does tranexamic acid stop haemoptysis? Interact Cardiovasc Thorac Surg. 2013;17(6):991–4.
39. Valipour A, Kreuzer A, Koller H, Koessler W, Burghuber OC. Bronchoscopy-guided topical hemostatic tamponade therapy for the management of life-threatening hemoptysis. Chest. 2005;127(6):2113–8.
40. Chung IH, Park MH, Kim DH, Jeon GS. Endobronchial stent insertion to manage hemoptysis caused by lung cancer. J Korean Med Sci. 2010;25(8):1253–5.
41. Dutau H, Palot A, Haas A, Decamps I, Durieux O. Endobronchial embolization with a silicone spigot as a temporary treatment for massive hemoptysis: a new bronchoscopic approach of the disease. Respiration. 2006;73(6):830–2.
42. Kho SS, Chan SK, Yong MC, Tie ST. Endobronchial embolization for life-threatening hemoptysis with Endobronchial Watanabe Spigot. BMC Res Notes. 2017;10(1):304.
43. Bolliger CT, Sutedja TG, Strausz J, Freitag L. Therapeutic bronchoscopy with immediate effect: laser, electrocautery, argon plasma coagulation and stents. Eur Respir J. 2006;27(6):1258–71.
44. Han CC, Prasetyo D, Wright GM. Endobronchial palliation using Nd:YAG laser is associated with improved survival when combined with multimodal adjuvant treatments. J Thorac Oncol. 2007;2(1):59–64.
45. Gershman E, Guthrie R, Swiatek K, Shojaee S. Management of hemoptysis in patients with lung cancer. Ann Transl Med. 2019;7(15):358.
46. Zenker M. Argon plasma coagulation. GMS Krankenhhyg Interdiszip. 2008;3(1):Doc15.
47. Cai J, Ribkoff J, Olson S, Raghunathan V, Al-Samkari H, DeLoughery TG, et al. The many roles of tranexamic acid: an overview of the clinical indications for TXA in medical and surgical patients. Eur J Haematol. 2020;104(2):79–87.
48. Alabdrabalnabi F, Alshahrani M, Ismail N. Nebulized tranexamic acid for recurring hemoptysis in critically ill patients: case series. Int J Emerg Med. 2020;13(1):45.
49. Klooster K, Slebos DJ. Endobronchial valves for the treatment of advanced emphysema. Chest. 2021;159(5):1833–42.
50. Lalla U, Allwood BW, Sinha Roy S, Irusen EM, Koegelenberg CFN. Endobronchial valve used as salvage therapy in a mechanically ventilated patient with intractable life-threatening haemoptysis. Respiration. 2017;93(6):436–40.
51. Mannucci PM. Desmopressin (DDAVP) in the treatment of bleeding disorders: the first 20 years. Blood. 1997;90(7):2515–21.
52. Squires JE. Indications for platelet transfusion in patients with thrombocytopenia. Blood Transfus. 2015;13(2):221–6.

12 Anesthesia for Pleural Interventions: Thoracentesis, Pleuroscopy, and Pleurodesis

Prarthna Chandar, Basvana Goudra, and Divakara Gouda

12.1 Introduction

Medical thoracoscopy, also referred to as pleuroscopy, is primarily employed as a diagnostic tool to examine the pleural space, although it also serves important therapeutic purposes [1]. Both symptomatic and asymptomatic recurrent exudative pleural effusions without a clear etiology after pleural fluid analysis represent the primary indication for diagnostic thoracoscopy. Chemical pleurodesis is the most common therapeutic indication for thoracoscopy, with other uses including therapeutic evacuation of effusions, deloculation of empyema, and endoscopic staging of mesothelioma [2].

Medical thoracoscopy has been in use for over a century, with the earliest descriptions involving the use of a cystoscope [3]. Today, it is performed as a minimally invasive procedure, typically under local anesthesia with or without sedation.

P. Chandar
Department of Pulmonology, Sidney Kimmel Medical College, Philadelphia, PA, USA
e-mail: Prarthna.Chandar@jefferson.edu

B. Goudra
Department of Anesthesiology, Sidney Kimmel Medical College, Jefferson Health, Philadelphia, PA, USA
e-mail: basavana.goudra@jefferson.edu

D. Gouda (✉)
PGY1, Internal Medicine, Inspira Health Network, Mullica Hill, NJ, USA
e-mail: goudad1@ihn.org

M. Sarkiss (ed.), *Anesthesia for Interventional Pulmonary Procedures*,
https://doi.org/10.1007/978-3-032-12007-6_12

12.2 Indications for Medical Thoracoscopy

While investigating pleural diseases, once pleural fluid analysis yields no definitive diagnosis, closed biopsy of the parietal pleura may be considered. Performed with or without ultrasound or CT guidance, closed biopsy is sometimes sufficient to diagnose conditions such as malignancy and pulmonary tuberculosis [4], though sensitivity and diagnostic yield for malignancies is very limited.. In contrast to closed pleural biopsy, medical thoracoscopy directly visualizes the pleura, and as a result, allows for targeted biopsy and, if necessary, therapeutic interventions. As a result, if available, medical thoracoscopy is the procedure of choice and is superior to closed pleural biopsy. Some of the indications for medical thoracoscopy include biopsy of the parietal pleura in patients with undiagnosed exudative pleural effusions, inserting a pleural catheter, performing pleural decortication in patients with stage 2 empyema, treating primary, secondary spontaneous, iatrogenic, and traumatic pneumothoraxes with, for example, talc poudrage [5], chemical pleurodesis with talc for recurrent hepatic hydrothorax [6], and treatment of chylothorax with fibrin sealant patch [7]. Those with primary spontaneous pneumothorax are generally young and are great surgical candidates as many will have bullae disease. As a result, VATS is generally preferred in this subgroup. Large-biopsy specimens can also obtained (for diagnosis as well as molecular testing of any cancer that has seeded to the pleural) to evaluate estrogen and progestin receptor expression in breast cancer and epidermal growth factor receptor expression in lung cancer [8].

12.3 Description of the Procedure

Both video-assisted thoracoscopic surgery (VATS) and medical thoracoscopy allow inspection of pleural space, obtainment of a tissue sample and therapeutic interventions. Unlike video-assisted thoracoscopic surgery that is performed with general anesthesia and endotracheal or endobronchial intubation, or single-lung ventilation, medical thoracoscopy is typically performed with moderate sedation and local infiltration. The latter procedure is usually performed in a bronchoscopy suite. Additionally, VATS also allows exploration of visceral pleura and typically involves 3–4 ports, while medical thoracoscopy utilizes 1 occasionally 2 ports (Fig. 12.1 and 12.2).

Once the patient is transported into the procedure room and connected to monitoring devices, lateral position is typically adapted, with the arm of that side abducted and secured above the head. Appropriate padding is necessary to protect all pressure points, including the elbow and between the legs. Placing a roll under the chest will assist in expanding the intercostal space. In general, patients who are diabetic, extremely thin or obese, use tobacco, or who have undergone surgery lasting more than 4 h are at increased risk for developing normally preventable peripheral nerve injuries [9]. Prior interventions in the same space such as pleurodesis or VATS, or radiotherapy in the area of interest increase the risk of injuries.

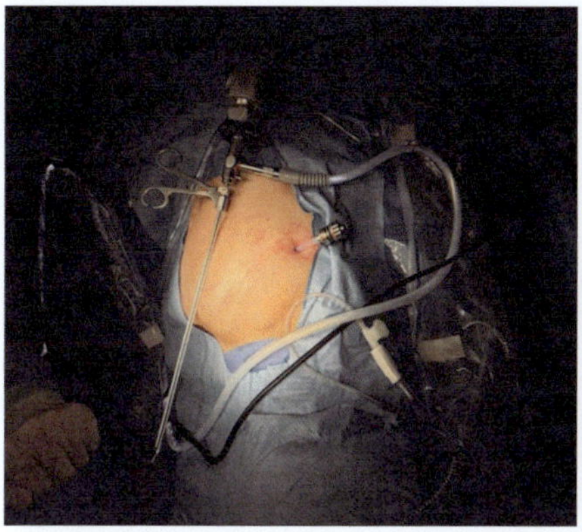
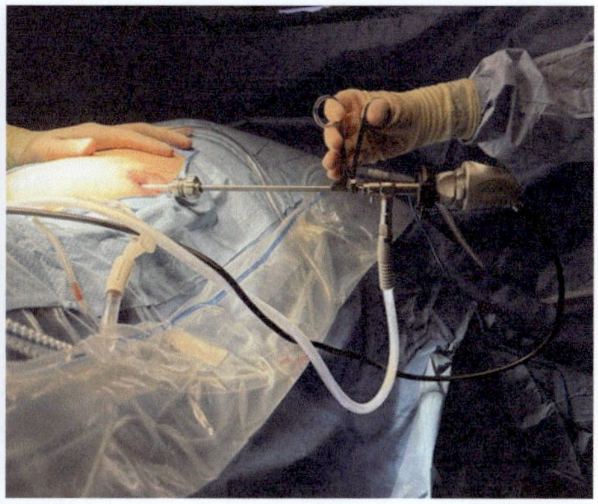

Figs. 12.1 and 12.2 Medical thoracoscopy procedure

Before the procedure, the pulmonologist typically repeats the ultrasound to determine the pathology and locate the appropriate site for thoracoscope insertion. The fifth intercostal space of the mid or anterior axillary line is the preferred site for port insertion.

12.4 Anesthetic Management

12.4.1 Preprocedure Assessment

In addition to standard preprocedure evaluation, system and pathology-specific evaluation is important. The most common indication for medical thoracoscopy is evaluation of pleural collections, typically when malignancy or tuberculosis is suspected. All measures to protect healthcare workers in the case of tuberculosis should be taken, the most important being personal protection with respirators [10]. If such measures are not implemented, such as when pulmonary tuberculosis is diagnosed after a procedure, those exposed need serial testing for latent TB infection.

Depending on the degree of pleural effusion, dyspnea is the most common symptom [11]. The mechanism of breathlessness is complicated and not strictly correlated with the degree of effusion. In fact, drainage of effusion is poorly correlated with symptom relief. Diaphragmatic function can be negatively affected after drainage, with an increase in compensatory drive. In spite of supplemental oxygen, these patients can desaturate quickly. The factors that contribute to such desaturation are ventilation-perfusion resulting from re-expansion of parts of the lung, re- expansion pulmonary edema, pneumothorax, and underlying pulmonary pathology. Administration of sedatives in addition to positioning, with the healthy lung dependent, further contributes to rapid decompensation. One can preempt such situations with adequate preparation and proactive measures such as use of a high-flow nasal cannula or non-rebreathing mask. Comorbidities such as increased age, underlying malignancy, and smoking history are additional factors that predispose to poor outcome [12].

12.4.2 Positioning, Monitoring, and Airway Devices

Patients are typically placed in lateral position, with the diseased side up. This is followed by placement of an ultrasound probe to locate a safe site for probe entry. The majority of patients are managed with standard monitoring as recommended by the American Society of Anesthesiologists [13]. In the event of conversion to general anesthesia, additional monitoring such as temperature is required. Invasive monitoring is normally not needed unless a patient is transferred from an intensive care unit with such monitoring in place. Obtaining an adequate end-tidal gas sample can be challenging when supplemental oxygen is delivered via high-flow nasal cannula.

Supplemental oxygen is typically administered with a standard nasal cannula. As explained, these patients are prone to desaturation. Both diaphragmatic excursions and compromised lung volumes resulting from pleural disease can compromise oxygen reserve and ventilation. Administration of sedatives will reduce respiratory drive, potentially causing dangerous hypoxia. An anesthesia provider should be prepared to support or control the airway and provide additional oxygenation as necessary.

Although there are no studies specifically evaluating the role of high-flow nasal cannula (HFNC) in the management of medical thoracoscopy, the device is extensively studied in similar procedures. These include patients undergoing gastrointestinal endoscopy, patients receiving ICU-level care, and post-thoracoscopic lobectomy [14–16]. Luo et al., in a retrospective data analysis, showed that the use of HFNC therapy can effectively reduce the incidence of $SpO_2 < 90\%$ during bronchoscopy in patients with hypoxemia, with an overall reduction in the incidence of adverse events [17]. Preparations should be always made to secure the airway with either a laryngeal mask airway or endotracheal tube.

12.4.3 Choice of Sedatives and Their Administration

In general, medical thoracoscopies are performed with moderate sedation, although the need and request for deep sedation have increased [18–21]. Propofol, midazolam, and fentanyl are few of the commonly employed sedatives in thoracoscopy. Other drugs studied in research settings and sparingly used in clinical practice are remifentanil, remimazolam, and dexmedetomidine.

The safety of propofol for medical thoracoscopy is well accepted. In a retrospective cohort study of patients who underwent pleuroscopy, the incidence of hypoxia defined as an oxygen saturation of less than 90% for 2 min was 4.5% (9/199 patients). The incidence of hypotension, another anticipated adverse event, was 38.2% (76/199) [21]. Avoidance of opioids reduced the incidence of hypoxia ($p = 0.021$) and improved mean oxygen saturations.

Grendelmeie et al. prospectively randomized 90 consecutive patients undergoing medical thoracoscopy into intravenous propofol and midazolam groups. Propofol, as expected, was associated with greater and more frequent hypoxia compared to midazolam. However, no procedure was aborted and none required an artificial airway, mechanical ventilation, or ICU-level care [19]. Use of the bispectral index as a depth of sedation monitor to titrate the administration of propofol and fentanyl was associated with hypoxemia [18]. Moderate sedation, typically with midazolam and fentanyl, with local infiltration, is typically administered by non-anesthesiologist providers under the supervision of a pulmonologist performing the procedure and found to be safe [22].

Among newer drugs, dexmedetomidine, an alpha-2 adrenergic agonist, was evaluated against midazolam, a short-acting benzodiazepine, for medical thoracoscopy. In this prospective pilot study, dexmedetomidine was found to be more efficacious than midazolam [23]. The need for fentanyl was less in patients receiving dexmedetomidine and with decreased coughing.

In practice, propofol is the hypnotic agent most commonly used for monitored anesthesia care (MAC), also known as deep sedation [24]. The use of fentanyl is usually necessary to provide a degree of analgesia with additional cough suppression. While moderate sedation allows purposeful response to verbal commands (alone or accompanied by light tactile stimulation), MAC typically provides deeper sedation. The physician performing the procedure usually supervises the administration of moderate sedation, while deep sedation is performed by an anesthesia provider. Propofol may be administered as an intermittent bolus. However, more commonly it is administered with an infusion pump, either as a continuous infusion or for a predetermined variable targeted plasma or brain concentration. The anesthesia provider supports the airway and circulation and ensures adequate oxygenation. Monitoring for any complications is essential. After the procedure, the anesthesia provider ensures return to near baseline status before transfer to recovery. Any deterioration or changes in status requires conversion to general anesthesia or lightening depth of sedation. Occasionally, patients require transfer to the ICU with or without respiratory support, including an endotracheal tube with mechanical ventilation or noninvasive ventilation.

12.4.4 Role of Regional Techniques

Local anesthetic medical thoracoscopy (LAT) is very popular in most parts of the world. Aujayeb and Jackson analyzed data from 275 patients who underwent LAT between January 2010 and December 2018. The procedure indications were malignant pleural mesothelioma, chronic inflammation/fibrinous pleuritis, lung cancer, and breast cancer. Of 275 patients, talcum pleurodesis was performed in 146 patients and was successful in 86%. It should be noted that, in addition to local anesthetic infiltration, all patients received conscious sedation with midazolam and fentanyl. Of note, the institution in which this study was performed later switched to patient-targeted anesthesia with propofol and remifentanil [25]. LAT is performed with a local anesthetic consisting typically of 20 mL of bupivacaine containing epinephrine (0.5% w/v, one in 200,000). This was injected into the selected intercostal space with the patient in the lateral decubitus position, following thoracic ultrasound to identify the optimal site for incision and port placement. Drainage of pleural effusion typically requires local anesthetic injection in the IV-V intercostal space along the midaxillary line [26]. Both rigid and semirigid thoracoscopes may be employed. A great narrative review provides detailed information about local anesthetic thoracoscopy indications, technical aspects, and complications in patients who present with unexplained pleural effusion with a high pre-test probability of cancer [27].

Paravertebral block is typically performed under ultrasound guidance and widely employed to provide postoperative analgesia in thoracic surgery [1]. Although rarely utilized during medical thoracoscopy, it offers pain relief comparable to that of thoracic epidural injections in patients undergoing cardiothoracic procedures. In a study by Agnoletti et al., paravertebral block was performed in 26 consecutive patients aged 18–90 years with ASA I–III undergoing elective medical thoracoscopy [2]. The procedure was carried out in either the lateral or sitting decubitus position by advancing a 22G Quincke spinal needle at thoracic (T) levels 3–7 until contact was made with the transverse process. From there, the needle was redirected approximately 1 cm off the transverse process to access the paravertebral space. Ropivacaine 1% (10 mg ml^{-1}) 2.5 ml and lidocaine 2% (20 mg ml^{-1}) 2.5 ml were used at each level. The procedures performed were therapeutic evacuation of pleural effusion, pleural biopsy, deloculation of empyema, and talc pleurodesis. Excellent hemodynamic stability with adequate analgesia was achieved.

Erector spinae plane block use for medical thoracoscopy is described by McPherson, Halvey, and ASujayeb [28]. In a pilot study, the technique was used on nine patients undergoing medical thoracoscopy. The procedure involves deposition of local anesthetic under ultrasound guidance within the fascial plane beneath the erector spinae muscles [29]. Spread of local anesthetic into the paravertebral space anesthetizes the thoracic spinal nerve roots. A single injection or sometimes two can cover multiple spinal levels. 20–35 mL of 0.25% l-bupivacaine was used for each injection by McPherson et al. Sedation was provided with propofol by anesthesia providers using a target-controlled infusion pump set to deliver a plasma concentration of 1.92 μg/mL along with remifentanil delivered to maintain a plasma concentration of 2.52 ng per mL. In addition to assisting the performance of the procedure, the block provides significant analgesia lasting several hours into the postprocedure period. Sharp et al. performed single injection erector spinae plane blocks on 26 patients and observed that average intraoperative and postoperative opioid consumption in oral morphine equivalents were 18.4 ± 15.8 and 11.2 ± 19.6 mg, respectively [30]. A single injection block was performed with 20 mL of 0.5% ropivacaine. Postoperative nausea and vomiting were not significant. Pain scores were similar between preoperative and postoperative periods.

There is insufficient research into the use of pectoral nerve and serratus anterior plane blocks during medical thoracoscopy. However, both blocks are used to provide postoperative pain relief after thoracoscopic lung surgeries.

12.5 Perioperative Complications and Their Management

Empyema, bleeding, port-site tumor growth, bronchopleural fistula, postoperative pneumothorax or air leak, pneumonia, and subcutaneous emphysema are some of the complications of medical thoracoscopy mentioned in the literature. There is an increased risk of infection in general, not just localized to lungs or site of the procedure including sepsis.

In a retrospective and prospective analysis of 127 patients undergoing medical thoracoscopy, Ahmed et al. documented prolonged air leak requiring long drainage (14/127), fever, lung laceration, hospital-acquired infection, and subcutaneous emphysema as some of the complications in that order of frequency [31]. Lung laceration was the most serious complication (3/127), and all occurred during the introduction of the trocar. They recommend active chest physiotherapy and early mobilization to reduce basal atelectasis and postprocedure infections. Although there were 11 deaths, none were related to postprocedure complications. Occasionally, trocar insertion can fail (2/127 in this series). The causes were presence of severe adhesions (causing obliteration of the pleural cavity) and hemopneumothorax due to the spontaneous rupture of an emphysematous bulla.

In another retrospective study involving 147 patients, 136 had pleural effusion and 11 had diffuse pulmonary infiltration [32]. They documented very low rate of complications (0.6%), including empyema, pleurocutaneous fistula, and transcutaneous growth of tumor (mesothelioma). Similarly, Brims et al. rarely documented any serious complications following medical thoracoscopy [33]. Six (6/58) patients experienced hospital-acquired infections, with all having malignancy. Persistent hydropneumothorax 5 days postprocedure occurred in 11/58 patients.

In a relatively larger retrospective study of 1926 patients from the People's Republic of China, 662 underwent diagnostic procedures, with the remaining undergoing therapeutic procedures [34]. Lung laceration was documented in six patients (0.3%). There was one death during the creation of artificial pneumothorax, deemed to be caused by air embolism or an inhibition of phrenic motoneurons and the circulatory system. While pain and fever were seen most often in patients who underwent pleurodesis, skin infection at the port of entry was reported most frequently in the pleural decortication of the empyema group.

12.6 Conclusions

Medical thoracoscopy is a safe procedure with a very high diagnostic yield, nearing 100 percent for malignancy and tuberculosis. Less frequently, it is employed for therapeutic procedures such as chemical pleurodesis. In North American clinical practice (including at the Thomas Jefferson University Hospital, Philadelphia), these procedures are generally performed under monitored anesthesia care (deep sedation), typically with propofol without resorting to any artificial airway such as endotracheal intubation or laryngeal mask airway. Standard monitoring is usually sufficient, and oxygenation can be adequately supported with supplementation using a nasal cannula. Local anesthetic administration or any of the many blocks discussed above will allow reduction of sedation and assist in postprocedural analgesia. Complications are rare, lung laceration being the most dangerous. Intraprocedural mortality is extremely rare.

References

1. Xu X, Xie YX, Zhang M, Du JH, He JX, Hu LH. Comparison of Thoracoscopy-guided thoracic paravertebral block and ultrasound-guided thoracic paravertebral block in postoperative analgesia of Thoracoscopic lung cancer radical surgery: a randomized controlled trial. Pain Ther. 2024;13(3):577–88.
2. Agnoletti V, Gurioli C, Piraccini E, Maitan S, Massimo Corso R, Matteo B, et al. Efficacy and safety of thoracic paravertebral block for medical thoracoscopy. Br J Anaesth. 2011;106(6):916–7.
3. Jacobaeus HV. Uber die Moglichkeit, die Zystoskopie bei Untersuchung seroser Hohlungen anzuwenden. Munch Med Wochenschr. 1910;40:2090–2.
4. Poe RH, Israel RH, Utell MJ, Hall WJ, Greenblatt DW, Kallay MC. Sensitivity, specificity, and predictive values of closed pleural biopsy. Arch Intern Med. 1984;144(2):325–8.
5. Fantin A, Castaldo N, Crisafulli E, Sartori G, Aujayeb A, Vailati P, et al. The role of medical Thoracoscopy with talc Poudrage in spontaneous, iatrogenic, and traumatic pneumothorax: a prolonged experience of a tertiary care center. Pulm Ther. 2024;10(3):347–62.
6. Rahim Y, Reddy RV, Naeem M, Tsaknis G. Medical thoracoscopy with talc pleurodesis for refractory hepatic hydrothorax: a case series of three successes. Respir Med Case Rep. 2024;50:102039.
7. Fiorelli A, Capasso F, Messina G, Natale G. Thoracoscopic management of chylothorax by application of a fibrin sealant patch. Heart Lung Circ. 2024;33(7):e35–7.
8. Michaud G, Berkowitz DM, Ernst A. Pleuroscopy for diagnosis and therapy for pleural effusions. Chest. 2010;138(5):1242–6.
9. Bouyer-Ferullo S. Preventing perioperative peripheral nerve injuries. AORN J. 2013;97(1):110–124.e9.
10. Diel R, Nienhaus A, Witte P, Ziegler R. Protection of healthcare workers against transmission of mycobacterium tuberculosis in hospitals: a review of the evidence. ERJ Open Res. 2020;6(1):00317–2019.
11. Muruganandan S, Mishra E, Singh B. Breathlessness with pleural effusion: what do we know? Semin Respir Crit Care Med. 2023;44(4):502–8.
12. Hinkelbein J, Lamperti M, Akeson J, Santos J, Costa J, De Robertis E, et al. European Society of Anaesthesiology and European Board of Anaesthesiology guidelines for procedural sedation and analgesia in adults. Eur J Anaesthesiol. 2018;35(1):6–24.
13. Standards for Basic Anesthetic Monitoring [Internet]. [cited 2025 Mar 28]. Available from: https://www.asahq.org/standards-and-practice-parameters/standards-for-basic-anesthetic-monitoring.
14. Goudra B, Gouda G, Singh PM. Recent developments in devices used for gastrointestinal endoscopy sedation. Clin Endosc. 2021;54(2):182–92.
15. Yu Y, Qian X, Liu C, Zhu C. Effect of high-flow nasal cannula versus conventional oxygen therapy for patients with Thoracoscopic lobectomy after Extubation. Can Respir J. 2017;2017:7894631.
16. Wittenstein J, Ball L, Pelosi P, Gama de Abreu M. High-flow nasal cannula oxygen therapy in patients undergoing thoracic surgery: current evidence and practice. Curr Opin Anaesthesiol. 2019;32(1):44–9.
17. Luo X, Xiang F. High-flow nasal cannula oxygen therapy versus conventional oxygen therapy in patients undergoing bronchoscopy: a retrospective study. BMC Pulm Med. 2024;24(1):614.

18. Tschopp JM, Purek L, Frey JG, Schnyder JM, Diaper J, Cartier V, et al. Titrated sedation with propofol for medical thoracoscopy: a feasibility and safety study. Respiration. 2011;82(5):451–7.
19. Grendelmeier P, Tamm M, Jahn K, Pflimlin E, Stolz D. Propofol versus midazolam in medical thoracoscopy: a randomized, noninferiority trial. Respir Int Rev Thorac Dis. 2014;88(2):126–36.
20. Vorster MJ, Bruwer JW, Frank W, Bernasconi M, Koegelenberg CF. The use of propofol for sedation in medical thoracoscopy. Respir Int Rev Thorac Dis. 2015;89(5):435.
21. Vakil E, Sarkiss M, Ost D, Vial MR, Casal RF, Eapen GA, et al. Safety of monitored anesthesia care using Propofol-based sedation for Pleuroscopy. Respiration. 2018;95(1):1–7.
22. Cohen NA, Stead SW. Moderate sedation for chest physicians. Chest. 2008;133(6):1489–94.
23. Sirohiya P, Kumar V, Mittal S, Gupta N, Garg R, Bharati SJ, et al. Dexmedetomidine versus midazolam for sedation during medical Thoracoscopy: a pilot randomized-controlled trial (RCT). J Bronchol Interv Pulmonol. 2022;29(4):248.
24. Statement on Distinguishing Monitored Anesthesia Care ("MAC") from Moderate Sedation/Analgesia (Conscious Sedation) [Internet]. [cited 2025 Mar 27]. Available from: https://www.asahq.org/standards-and-practice-parameters/statement-on-distinguishing-monitored-anesthesia-care-from-moderate-sedation-analgesia.
25. Aujayeb A, Jackson K. A review of the outcomes of rigid medical thoracoscopy in a large UK district general hospital. Pleura Peritoneum. 2020;5(4):20200131.
26. Bodtger U, Porcel JM, Bhatnagar R, Maskell N, Munavvar M, Jensen C, et al. Local anesthetic thoracoscopy for undiagnosed pleural effusion. J Vis Exp. 2023;201:e65734.
27. Piazzolla M, De Pace CC, Porcel JM, Tondo P. Local anesthetic Thoracoscopy: a focus on indications, Techniques and Complications. Arch Bronconeumol. 2024;60(7):423–30.
28. McPherson J, Halvey E, Aujayeb A. Erector spinae plane blocks for day-case medical thoracoscopy: a pilot clinical study. Pleura Peritoneum. 2022;7(4):187–90.
29. Forero M, Adhikary SD, Lopez H, Tsui C, Chin KJ. The erector Spinae plane block: a novel analgesic technique in thoracic neuropathic pain. Reg Anesth Pain Med. 2016;41(5):621–7.
30. Sharp A, Mudda G, Braehler MR, Gesthalter YB. Erector Spinae plane block: a novel anesthetic approach for Pleuroscopy. J Bronchol Interv Pulmonol. 2022;29(2):109–14.
31. Nour Moursi Ahmed S, Saka H, Mohammadien HA, Alkady O, Oki M, Tanikawa Y, et al. Safety and complications of medical Thoracoscopy. Adv Med. 2016;2016:3794791.
32. Hansen M, Faurschou P, Clementsen P. Medical thoracoscopy, results and complications in 146 patients: a retrospective study. Respir Med. 1998;92(2):228–32.
33. Brims FJH, Arif M, Chauhan AJ. Outcomes and complications following medical thoracoscopy. Clin Respir J. 2012;6(3):144–9.
34. Wan YY, Zhai CC, Lin XS, Yao ZH, Liu QH, Zhu L, et al. Safety and complications of medical thoracoscopy in the management of pleural diseases. BMC Pulm Med. 2019;19:125.

The Bronchoscopy Suite

13

Mona Sarkiss

13.1 Introduction

It was December 2002 when I was first asked by the anesthesia department leadership at MD Anderson Cancer Center to investigate providing anesthesia support in a bronchoscopy suite outside the operating room environment. At that time, I was not able to find any precedents to such setup. Other large academic institutions were performing bronchoscopic procedures requiring anesthesia support mostly in the operating room. General skepticism among the anesthesia faculty about the safety of performing airway procedures under general anesthesia outside the operating room was prevalent. My first visit to the bronchoscopy suite added to the concerns expressed by other faculty members regarding the remoteness from the operating room and the limited space available to add the needed anesthesia equipment and supplies. I began by making a list of what is needed to establish a safe anesthesia service in what I believed to be one of the first out of the operating room bronchoscopy suite with anesthesia support in the United States. In this chapter, I will describe my learning journey complemented with the current literature on how to set up a bronchoscopy suite and establish a safe anesthesia practice for interventional bronchoscopy/pulmonology procedures.

13.2 The Bronchoscopy Suite Versus the Operating Room

The first question interventional pulmonologists encounter when they request anesthesia support in a bronchoscopy suite is: why not perform the procedures in the operating room? The argument is that the operating room with its trained staff

M. Sarkiss (✉)
Department of Anesthesiology and Perioperative Medicine, Department of Pulmonary Medicine, The University of Texas MD Anderson Cancer Canter, Houston, TX, USA
e-mail: msarkiss@mdanderson.org

M. Sarkiss (ed.), *Anesthesia for Interventional Pulmonary Procedures*,
https://doi.org/10.1007/978-3-032-12007-6_13

anesthesiologist, emergency equipment, and the additional support staff in the event of emergency is best suited for airway procedures. Even though this argument was sound, there were multiple counterarguments that led us to consider establishing anesthesia services in the bronchoscopy suite outside the operating room [1]. The first and foremost counterpoint was the lack of availability of a block time designated for interventional pulmonary procedure in the busy operating room schedule. Interventional bronchoscopic procedures would generally be placed on hold until an operating room with support staff becomes available. Alternatively, the procedures would be scheduled as an emergency add-on to the schedule of the day. These arrangements made it clear that having procedures scheduled and performed on a daily and/or emergency basis would be difficult and unattainable. In some institutions, the interventional pulmonologists are granted 1 or 2 days per week when they can schedule their procedures in the operating room. Even though these agreements allowed the interventional pulmonologists to perform their procedures on weekly basis, it did not give room for growth with the increasing demand for bronchoscopic intervention to diagnose and treat central and peripheral airway/pulmonary disease. Additionally, limiting the practice to 1 or 2 days per week hindered the interventional pulmonologist's ability to perform emergency cases needing immediate care such as critical central airway obstruction or acute massive hemoptysis. Having a designated bronchoscopy suite with complete anesthesia care on a daily basis at multiple institutions enhanced the growth of the interventional pulmonary practice and allowed for emergency add-on as needed [1, 2].

Efficiency of care was the second main counterpoint to performing interventional pulmonary procedures in the operating room. As the field of interventional pulmonology grew over the years, the number, size, and sophistication of equipment needed increased [3]. For example, the endobronchial ultrasound bronchoscope and the processor needed to store the image, the robotic bronchoscope supported with confocal CT scanner, and different sizes of flexible and rigid bronchoscopes needed are a few of the large-size equipment requiring storage space and ability to transport to the operating room safely each time a case is scheduled. Once the equipment is transferred to the operating room, additional work and time are needed to reconnect the equipment to the computer processors that creates and stores images taken during the procedure. At the end of the procedure, a reverse process of disassembling all the used equipment and transferring it back to its cleaning and/or storage location is required. The frequent transport, assembly, and disassembly of large and small equipment needed for interventional bronchoscopy are associated with extra time wasted, damage to the valuable equipment, and extra cost to repair the damaged equipment. A procedure that could be completed in 1 h would take double or triple the time with the additional unanticipated cost for repairs.

Lastly, the counterpoint of financial stewardship [3]. The cost of the procedure incurred to both the hospital and the patient, especially in relation to the revenue gained in return, should be considered. A simple business plan can be created to calculate the cost of the utilization of an operating room for 1–2 h per procedure, payments to the OR personnel involved in the procedure (technicians, nursing, nursing aid), and the anesthesia services and supplies in the OR versus providing the same service in the bronchoscopy suite. The cost should then be compared to the revenue paid by a mix of insurance companies and self-payors. The cost to both the patient and the hospital when a procedure is performed in the operating room vs. the bronchoscopy suite can be displayed side by side, making for a strong argument that procedures performed in the bronchoscopy suite would cut the cost to both the patient and the hospital while generating a higher revenue. The main question then becomes how to provide financially sound interventional bronchoscopic procedures in the bronchoscopy suite with the same level of quality of care provided in the operating room. This leads us to the next section describing the setup of anesthesia support in the bronchoscopy suite that ensure safe anesthesia care equivalent to that provided in the OR.

13.3 The Bronchoscopy Suite Design

The overall goal of designing a bronchoscopy suite is to create a replica of an operating room with a setup for anesthesia support. It is essential to have all safety protocols, supplies for emergencies and comprehensive preprocedure, and postprocedure care included within the suite design [4].

13.3.1 The Bronchoscopy Suite Layout

The common layout of an operating room is where the anesthesia staff, anesthesia machine, supplies cart, and medication dispensing cart are located at the head of the bed. This location designation was based on the role and responsibility of the anesthesia staff to manage the airway and maintain its patency during surgery. In the bronchoscopy suite, the airway management is shared between the anesthesiologist and the interventional pulmonologist, making such arrangement impractical, as both the anesthesia and interventional pulmonology staff and equipment will be crowded at the head of the bed. Such tight space sharing can cause difficulty in maneuvering while managing the airway and/or performing the procedure and even unsafe during emergencies.

For the abovementioned reason, a different layout of the bronchoscopy suite had to be considered. The current layout at the MD Anderson Cancer Center has the proceduralist and the bronchoscopy equipment (flexible, rigid, and robot) stationed at the head of the bed. The procedure's monitors hang from a boom at the foot of the bed making the monitors in direct vision of the proceduralist. The anesthesia machine and the anesthesia monitor are stationed at the foot of the bed where the anesthesia monitor is aligned with the bronchoscopy monitor (Fig. 13.1). This alignment enables the proceduralist to see both the patient's vital signs and the bronchoscopy images side by side during the procedure (Fig. 13.2). The anesthesia staff work area is at the right side of the patient's bed with ample space for the supplies cart and medication dispensing cart. Most importantly, the anesthesia work area location enables the anesthesia staff to visualize both the patient's vital signs and the

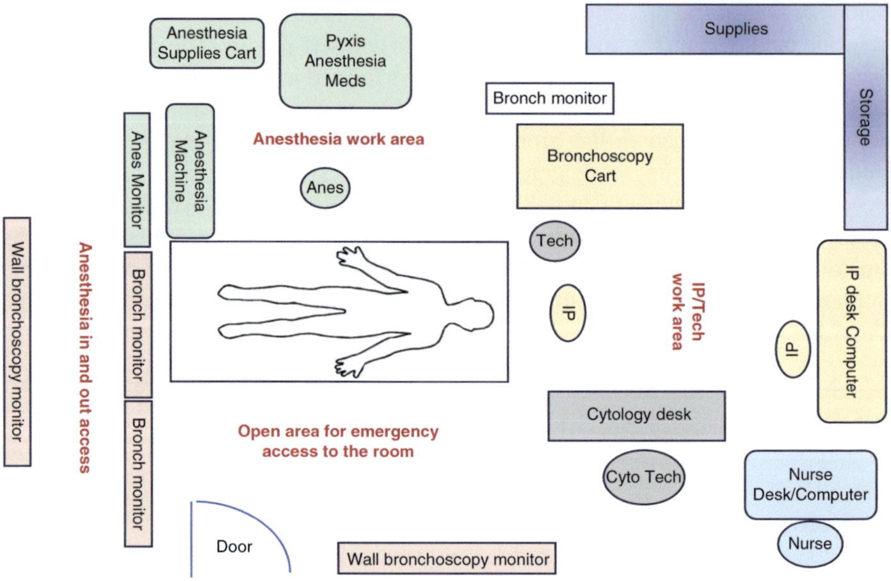

Fig. 13.1 The configuration of the bronchoscopy suite

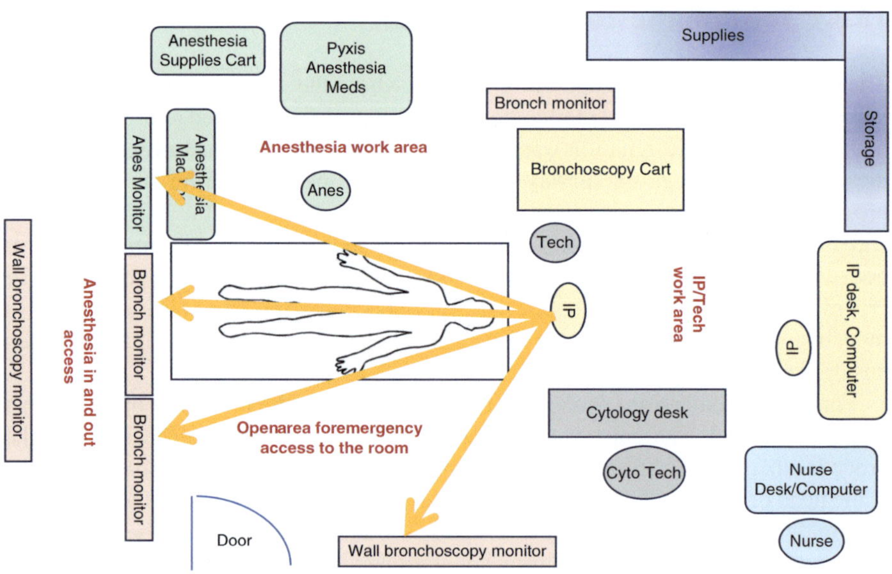

Fig. 13.2 The field of vision for the proceduralist

progress of the procedure on the aligned bronchoscopy and anesthesia monitor screens (Fig. 13.3). The ability of both the anesthesiologist and the proceduralist to see the patient's vital and the bronchoscopy images side by side is vital in keeping clear communication throughout the procedure. Nursing staff and cytology technician are located to the left of the patient's bed, giving them easy access in and out of the procedure area to deliver samples to the onsite pathologist (Fig. 13.1). The open space between the patient's bed and the door is intentionally left open to facilitate the entrance of transport bed in and out of the procedure room in case of an emergency requiring rapid transfer to the operating room (Fig. 13.1).

Based on the above-described bronchoscopy suite setup, the anesthesiologist assisted by the nurse anesthetist can induce the anesthesia and manage the airway at the head of the bed. Once the airway is secured or after anesthesia induction for rigid bronchoscopy, the airway is handed over the proceduralist at the head of the bed and the anesthesia staff move to the right side of the bed where they can continue to monitor the patient and the progress of the procedure as well as manage the ventilator and administer medications as needed.

13.3.2 Anesthesia Equipment

The equipment can be divided into basic anesthesia supplies and those needed for emergencies [2].

The basic supplies include

- A compact anesthesia machine with volatile anesthetic. Sevoflurane has a potent bronchodilator effect that can be valuable if the patient suffers bronchospasm during the procedure. The compact ventilator is essential due to the

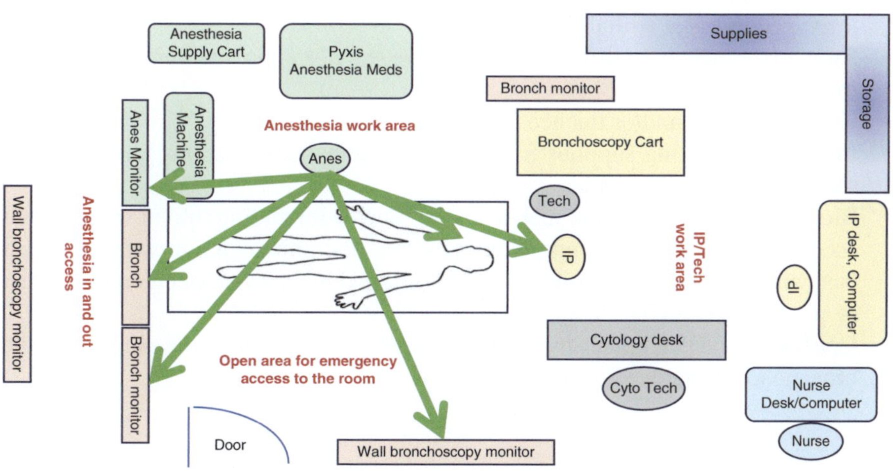

Fig. 13.3 The anesthesiologist field of vision

limited space in the out-of-operating room locations and facilitate repositioning the ventilator to other locations within the room based on the procedure performed. For example, during a pleuroscopy procedure the ventilator has to be angled away from the patient's bed to create space for the interventionalist and his/her assistants to stand at the sides of the bed to access the chest cavity during the procedure.

- Central wall supply and cylinders of oxygen and air. The air supply is essential when low FiO_2 is needed during thermal therapy.
- Wall suction and scavenging system to minimize room air contamination by the volatile anesthetic.
- Medication dispensing cart is needed especially if the bronchoscopy suite is located far from the pharmacy. However, the ability to rapidly communicate with the central pharmacy to promptly provide additional uncommon medications that may be needed during emergency is essential.
- Anesthesia supply cart that contains the needed supplies for IV placement, intubation, IV tubing, nasogastric tubes, arterial line setup, syringes, needles, etc.
- A designated cabinet for larger commonly used anesthesia supplies such as anesthesia circuits, Soda sorb, anesthesia masks, face masks and cannulas, and supraglottic airway devices of different sizes.
- A computer with stable intranet/Internet connectivity to be able to use the anesthesia electronic medical health record and have access to medical protocols and queries as needed.

The emergency supplies include

- Difficult airway supplies such as video laryngoscope devices, bougie, cook catheter, and Aintree catheter. However, when difficulty is encountered in intubation, the flexible bronchoscopes used for the interventional pulmonary procedure are readily available and the expertise of the pulmonologist in bronchoscopy can be leveraged to assist with the intubation.
- Bronchial blockers of different sizes can be stored by the interventional team or by the anesthesia team.
- Cricothyrotomy and/or tracheostomy kits.
- Invasive monitoring supplies for arterial line and central venous lines insertion should be readily available.
- Blood transfusion supplies such as blood transfusion tubing, blood warmer, and access to rapid infusion unit. A quick access to communication with the blood bank and a protocol for prompt delivery of blood in the event of emergency must be put in place.
- Crash cart and malignant hyperthermia cart must be within the vicinity of the bronchoscopy suite.

13.3.3 Preoperative and Postoperative Recovery Areas

It is essential to have designated preoperative and postoperative recovery areas within the bronchoscopy suite. The size of the space required and number of patients' beds within the recovery area should be based on the number of cases performed per day and the duration of the procedures as it relates to the proposed recovery time. This arrangement should allow for patients to have adequate time to recover and be discharged while others are undergoing the procedure without overcrowding and delays in transport from the procedure room to the recovery area. Additionally, the recovery area should follow the same hospital's standards and policies used for postoperative recovery in the main operating room suite.

13.3.4 Hazards

The work environment of the bronchoscopy suite can cause exposure to several health hazards. Understanding the risks and having protective protocols in place are essential for the safety of the personnel and patients in the bronchoscopy suite. These hazards include.

Infection Flexible and rigid bronchoscopy are considered aerosol-generating procedures. Therefore, all bronchoscopic procedures must be performed in a negative-pressure room to prevent the spread of airborne infection [1]. The air flows into the bronchoscopy suite from the outside and is suctioned out through a special vent to the outside of the hospital to prevent infecting staff and other patients [4]. However, during a pleuroscopy procedure, the bronchoscopy room needs to have positive pressure to prevent contaminants from the rest of the hospital air from infecting the patient undergoing the procedure similar to the conditions required in an operating room. Two separate ventilation systems are needed to switch between negative and positive pressure air flow as needed. Personal protective equipment and gear such as face masks, gowns, N-95 masks, and gloves should be readily available, and the hospital protocols for their usage in aerosol-producing procedures should be followed [5, 6].

Fire Thermal therapy is commonly used for the management of patients with central airway obstruction and/or hemoptysis, for example, argon plasma coagulation (APC), electrocautery, and laser. The combination of thermal energy, oxygen, and a substrate that can ignite can lead to airway, drapes, or even a patient's fire [5]. Care should be taken to lower the FiO_2 to $<40\%$ during thermal therapy or laser utilization and avoid insufflation of oxygen below the patient's draped when thermal energy source is in use.

Laser Therapy Commonly used during central airway canalization and management of bleeding from the airway mucosal surface. Protective eye wear and education regarding laser safety and appropriate handling of the Laser equipment must be undertaken. Additionally, lowering the FiO_2 during laser therapy is essential to prevent airway fires [5].

Radiation Exposure is encountered during procedures requiring fluoroscopy such as transbronchial lung biopsies or mobile cone-beam CT scanner used during robotic bronchoscopy [7]. Protective eye wear and lead apron with thyroid shields as well as personnel training on how to maintain personal safety during radiation exposure are essential [1, 4].

Room Air Contamination by Volatile Anesthetics Most bronchoscopic procedures are performed under total intravenous anesthesia to intentionally avoid the use of volatile anesthetics. Frequent opening of the airway devices during the insertion and the removal of the bronchoscope can lead to escape of volatile anesthetics and contamination of the bronchoscopy suite room air. Having a scavenging system connected to the anesthesia machine is essential to minimize personnel exposure to volatile anesthetics if its use is needed during the procedure [5].

References

1. Prakash UBS. Bronchoscopy unit, expertise, equipment and personnel. In: Mathur CTBPN, editor. Interventional bronchoscopy. 30. Progress in respiratory research. S.Karger AG; 1999. p. 31–43.
2. Abdelmalak BB, Gildea TR, Doyle DJ, Mehta AC. A blueprint for success: a multidisciplinary approach to clinical operations within a bronchoscopy suite. Chest. 2022;161(4):1112–21.
3. Amat BPR G, Agustí C, Xaubet A, Torres A. What is an interventional pulmonology unit in Europe? Clin Pulm Med. 2010;17(1):42–6.
4. Mehta AC, Avasarala SK, Jain P, Deshwal H, Gildea TR. A blueprint for success: design and implementation of an ideal bronchoscopy suite. Chest. 2020;157(3):712–23.
5. Chen K, Bai C. Occupational adverse effects and protective factors in bronchoscopy. J Thorac Dis. 2019;11(4):1651–61.
6. Culver DA, Gordon SM, Mehta AC. Infection control in the bronchoscopy suite: a review of outbreaks and guidelines for prevention. Am J Respir Crit Care Med. 2003;167(8):1050–6.
7. Tsai WS, Haywood E, Li X, Rosenbaum J, Lindsey B. Radiation in the bronchoscopy suite: one center's experience with navigational bronchoscopy and a review of the literature. J Bronchol Interv Pulmonol. 2025;32(2):e1001.

Recovery and Monitoring Postbronchoscopic Procedures

14

Ursula Galway and Basem Abdelmalak

14.1 Introduction

Bronchoscopic procedures may be performed under moderate or deep sedation or under general anesthesia. There is a trend to using general anesthesia for the more invasive and lengthier diagnostic and therapeutic bronchoscopic procedures. Bronchoscopic procedures are often performed on an outpatient basis and tend not to confer the same degree of pain or limitation that occurs postsurgical procedure; nonetheless, recovery requires the same postoperative care as any other surgical procedure regardless of the anesthetic technique or depth. Patients are often discharged on the same day; thus, it is preferable to use short-acting anesthetics that lessens the incidence of postoperative nausea and vomiting (PONV) and postprocedure sedation to achieve prompt discharge. Patients should be transported to a standard post anesthesia care unit (PACU) that can provide both phase 1 and 2 care. Patients should be monitored with standard monitors and supplemental oxygen provided if needed.

Postanesthesia care is divided into two phases. Phase 1 is the immediate post-general anesthesia care. Phase 1 requires close monitoring, including hemodynamics, pain control, fluid management, and the availability of support for positive pressure ventilation as needed. Phase 1 ends with full recovery from general anesthesia and return of vital signs to near baseline.

Postanesthesia phase 2 occurs after phase 1 and is the period of preparation for care at home or extended care environment and includes education, postop instructions, and prescribed discharge medication (street readiness) [1]. Due to the short-acting nature of the general anesthetics often used for bronchoscopic procedures,

U. Galway
Department of General Anesthesiology, Cleveland Clinic, Cleveland, OH, USA
e-mail: galwayu@ccf.org

B. Abdelmalak (✉)
Anesthesiology Institute, Cleveland Clinic Foundation, Cleveland, OH, USA
e-mail: abdelmb@ccf.org

M. Sarkiss (ed.), *Anesthesia for Interventional Pulmonary Procedures*,
https://doi.org/10.1007/978-3-032-12007-6_14

patients frequently proceed to phase 2 recovery quickly and rapidly meet PACU discharge criteria, often in 30–45 min.

The American Society of Anesthesiologists (ASA) delineates clear guidelines for postanesthesia care that are clearly stated in Table 14.1 [2].

Perioperative and postanesthetic management of the patient includes periodic assessment and monitoring of the following:

Table 14.1 PACU patient assessment and monitoring [2]

I. Patient assessment and monitoring
Periodic assessment of airway patency, respiratory rate, and oxygen saturation should be done during emergence and recovery
Particular attention should be given to monitoring oxygenation and ventilation
Routine monitoring of pulse and blood pressure should be done during emergence and recovery, and electrocardiographic monitors should be immediately available
Assessment of neuromuscular function should be performed during emergence and recovery for patients who have received nondepolarizing neuromuscular blocking agents or who have medical conditions associated with neuromuscular dysfunction
Mental status should be periodically assessed during emergence and recovery
Patient temperature should be periodically assessed during emergence and recovery
Pain should be periodically assessed during emergence and recovery
Periodic assessment of nausea and vomiting should be performed routinely during emergence and recovery
Postoperative hydration status should be assessed in the postanesthesia care unit and managed accordingly
Certain procedures involving significant loss of blood or fluids may require additional fluid management
Assessment of urine output and of urinary voiding should be done on a case-by-case basis for selected patients or selected procedures during emergence and recovery
Assessment of drainage and bleeding should be performed
II. Prophylaxis and treatment of nausea and vomiting
Antiemetic agents should be used for the prevention and treatment of nausea and vomiting when indicated
Multiple antiemetic agents may be used for the prevention or treatment of nausea and vomiting when indicated
III. Treatment during emergence and recovery
Administering supplemental oxygen during transportation or in the recovery room should be done for patients at risk of hypoxemia
Normothermia should be a goal during emergence and recovery
When available, forced air warming systems should be used for treating hypothermia
Meperidine should be used for the treatment of patient shivering during emergence and recovery when clinically indicated
Hypothermia, a common cause of shivering, should be treated by rewarming
Practitioners may consider other opioid agonists or agonists–antagonists when meperidine is contraindicated or not available
IV. Antagonism of the effects of sedatives, analgesics, and neuromuscular blocking agents
Specific antagonists should be available whenever benzodiazepines are administered
Flumazenil should not be used routinely but may be administered to antagonize respiratory depression and sedation in selected patients
After pharmacologic antagonism, patients should be observed long enough to ensure that cardiorespiratory depression does not recur

(continued)

Table 14.1 (continued)

Specific antagonists should be available whenever opioids are administered Opioid antagonists (e.g., naloxone) should not be used routinely but may be administered to antagonize respiratory depression in selected patients After pharmacologic antagonism, patients should be observed long enough to ensure that cardiorespiratory depression does not recur The Task Force reminds practitioners that acute antagonism of the effects of opioids may result in pain, hypertension, tachycardia, or pulmonary edema
Specific antagonists should be administered for reversal of residual neuromuscular blockade when indicated
V. *Protocol for discharge*
1. The routine requirement for urination before discharge should not be part of a discharge protocol and may only be necessary for selected patients
2. The requirement of drinking clear fluids should not be part of a discharge protocol and may only be necessary for selected patients, determined on a case-by-case basis (e.g., diabetic patients)
3. As part of a recovery room discharge protocol, all patients should be required to have a responsible individual accompany them home
4. Patients should be observed until they are no longer at increased risk for cardiorespiratory depression A *mandatory* minimum stay should not be required Discharge criteria should be designed to minimize the risk of central nervous system or cardiorespiratory depression after discharge

- Cardiovascular function (monitoring of pulse and blood pressure and availability of electrocardiographic monitors).
- Respiratory function (airway patency, respiratory rate, ventilation, and oxygen saturation).
- Patient temperature.
- Mental status.
- Neuromuscular function.
- Periodic assessment of nausea and vomiting and pain.
- Periodic assessment of drainage and bleeding.
- Postoperative hydration status.
- Urine output and of urinary voiding, which should be done on a case-by-case basis for selected patients or selected procedures. This is often not applicable in bronchoscopic procedures.

14.2 Recovery Room Standards

14.2.1 Standard for Vital Sign Frequency in Phases 1 and 2

The frequency of adult vital signs is institution specific, with frequency ranging from every 5 to 15 min. Vital signs should occur at a minimum on admission to the recovery room and then every 15 min during phase 1, and more frequently if needed as the clinical condition requires. At our institution, the policy is to monitor vitals every 15 min times 4 and then every 30 min times 2 followed by hourly while the patient is in phase 1. Phase 2 vital signs should be obtained upon admission and every 30–60 min or more frequently as needed per the patient's clinical status. Telemetry is frequently not performed in phase 2. Clinical judgment is the essential element in determining the frequency of vital signs [3]. For example, if the patient is alert and seems to be ready for discharge, then a full assessment including vital signs is performed regardless of when the prior assessment was done to assess for discharge readiness according to the discharge criteria [4].

14.2.2 Nursing Concurrency

ASPAN recommends that a nurse care for only one patient from the time the patient is first admitted until he or she is hemodynamically stable. Critical elements that need to be met before transitioning to a 1:2 ratio include

- Report has been received from the anesthesia care provider, questions answered, and the transfer of care has taken place.
- Patient has a stable/secure airway.
- Patient is hemodynamically stable.
- Patient is free from agitation, restlessness, and combative behaviors.
- Initial assessment is complete.

Patients should remain at a 1:1 nursing care ratio if there is any airway and/or hemodynamic instability, any unconscious patient 8 years of age and under, and patients with isolation precautions until there is sufficient time for donning and removing personal protective equipment (PPE) in these scenarios. A second nurse must be available to assist as necessary.

A 1:2 nurse–patient ratio in phase 1 allows for appropriate assessment, planning, implementation, and evaluation for discharge as well as increased efficiency and flow of patients through the phase 1 area. A 1:2 ratio may occur if there are.

- Two conscious patients, stable and free of complications, but not yet meeting discharge criteria.
- Two conscious patients, stable and under the age of 8 years, with family or competent support team members present, but not yet meeting discharge criteria [3].

A 1:3 nurse–patient ratio allows for appropriate assessment, planning, implementing care, and evaluation for discharge, as well as increasing efficiency and flow of patients through phase 2 [5].

14.2.3 Oxygen Delivery

Supplemental oxygen during transportation or in the recovery room should be administered for patients at risk of hypoxemia. While it is not necessary, supplemental oxygen should be considered in patients undergoing bronchoscopic procedures as they often have underlying pulmonary disease and may be at a higher risk of hypoxemia postprocedurally.

14.2.4 Voiding and Drinking

The routine requirement for urination before discharge should not be part of a discharge protocol and may only be necessary for selected patients such as patients receiving gynecological and urological surgery. This is not the case in bronchoscopic procedures, thus voiding is not a prerequisite to discharge in the bronchoscopy suite.

The requirement of drinking clear fluids should not be part of a discharge protocol and may only be necessary for selected patients, determined on a case-by-case basis (e.g., diabetic patients).

14.3 Recovery and Discharge Criteria

Discharge criteria are designed to determine a patient's readiness to safely leave the postanesthesia care unit. A PACU scoring system allows a safe, reliable, and reproducible discharge of patients after anesthesia. There are multiple variations of discharge criteria available.

Several scoring systems have been developed, both for the phase 1 and 2 PACU period. Some of the commonly used PACU scoring systems include the Aldrete Score, Modified Aldrete score, and the postanesthesia discharge scoring system (PADSS) [6–8] (Tables 14.2, 14.3 and 14.4).

Recovery criteria in general should be standardized and not time based, but based on clinical parameters [4]. The older criteria initially proposed in the 1970s were more suitable for discharging patients from PACU to the hospital floors. The original Aldrete score was modified as more objective data became available, that is, pulse ox [6]. The Modified Aldrete system includes five additional elements that are particularly useful during the phase 2 recovery period prior to discharge to home (dressing, pain, ambulation, feeding, urine output). It does not rely on subjective data from the original score such as color, but lacks nausea as a goal [7].

These scoring tools have undergone multiple revisions, with more recent versions focusing on ensuring that the patient is "street fit" before discharge. Such scoring tools provide a score based on clinical milestones to ensure safety and at the same time improve efficiency by discharging patients when they achieve an acceptable and safe score regardless of time spent in PACU. This score encompasses items such as level of consciousness, vital signs, physical activity, oxygen saturation, pain, nausea, and bleeding [4]. One such scoring system is the postanesthetic discharge scoring system (PADSS) [8]. This scoring system is based on vital signs, activity level, nausea or vomiting, pain, surgical bleeding, and intake and output; the criteria for discharge to home typically include a PADSS score $\geq$9. It was developed to give a home readiness discharge criterion for the ambulatory surgery setting. A

Table 14.2 Aldrete score, which includes five elements (activity, respiration, circulation, consciousness, oxygen saturation) [6]

Aldrete score 0–2 points assigned per component	
Activity	
Moves all 4 extremities	2
Moves 2 extremities	1
Unable to move any extremity	0
Respiration	
Able to deep breath and cough freely	2
Dyspnea, shallow or limited breathing	1
Apnea	0
Circulation	
SBP ± 20 mm Hg of preanesthetic level	2
SBP +20–50 mm Hg of preanesthetic level	1
SBP +50 mm Hg of preanesthetic level	0
Level of consciousness	
Alert	2
Drowsy by reusable on calling	1
No response	0
Color	
Normal	2
Pale or dusky	1
Cyanotic	0
Requirement for discharge criteria out of 10 points	*>9*

Table 14.3 Modified Aldrete score [7]

Variable	Assessment interpretation	Score
Activity	Able to move all extremities voluntarily or on command	2
	Able to move two extremities voluntarily or on command	1
	Unable to move extremities voluntarily or on command	0
Respiration	Able to breathe deeply and cough freely	2
	Dyspnea or limited breathing	1
	Apneic or on a mechanical ventilator	0
Circulation	Blood pressure +/– 20% or less of the preanesthetic level	2
	Blood pressure +/– 20% to 49% of the preanesthetic level	1
	Blood pressure +/– 50% or more of the preanesthetic level	0
Consciousness	Fully awake	2
	Arousable on calling	1
	Not responding	0
Oxygenation	Able to maintain O_2 saturation > 92% on room air	2
	Needs supplemental O_2 to maintain O_2 saturation > 90%	1
	O_2 saturation <90% even with supplemental oxygen	0

(continued)

Table 14.3 (continued)

Variable	Assessment interpretation	Score
Dressing	Dry and clean	2
	Wet but marked and not increasing	1
	A growing area of wetness	0
Pain	No pain	2
	Mild pain handled by oral medication	1
	Severe pain requiring parenteral medication	0
Ambulation	Able to stand up and walk straight	2
	Vertigo when erect	1
	Dizziness when supine	0
Fast-feeding	Able to drink fluids	2
	Nauseated	1
	Nausea and vomiting	0
Urine output	Has voided	2
	Unable to void but comfortable	1
	Unable to void and uncomfortable	0

Table 14.4 Postanesthesia discharge scoring system (PADSS) [9]

Vital signs	
Vital signs must be stable and consistent with age and preoperative baseline	
Blood pressure and pulse within 20% of baseline	2
BP and pulse within 20–40% of baseline	1
BP and pulse >40% of baseline	0
Activity level	
Patient must be able to ambulate at preoperative level	
Steady gait to dizziness, or meets preop level	2
Requires assistance	1
Unable to ambulate	0
Nausea and vomiting	
Patient should have minimal nausea and vomiting before discharge	
Minimal: successfully treated with or without	
Medication	2
Moderate: successfully treated with IM medication	1
Severe: continues after repeated treatment	0
Pain	
Patient should have minimal or no pain before discharge	
Level of pain that the patient has should be acceptable to the patient	
Pain acceptable	2
Pain not acceptable	1
Surgical bleeding	
Postsurgical bleeding should be consistent with expected blood loss for the procedure	
Minimal: does not require dressing change	2
Moderate: up to two dressing changes required	1
Severe: more than three dressing changes required	0
Requirement for discharge criteria out of 10 points	*>9*
PADSS should provide early recognition of patients in the ambulatory setting that will require prolonged or overnight observation of the patient for pain control, excess bleeding from the procedure or management of nausea and vomiting; this should prevent unexpected ER visits or return to hospital visits	

Table 14.5 Cleveland Clinic phase 2 discharge tool

Phase 2 discharge scoring tool
Level of consciousness
2 = fully awake
1 = arousable with verbal or tactile stimulation
0 = unresponsive
Physical activity (return to preanesthetic level)
2 = steady gait, no dizziness, or meets preop level
1 = requires assistance
0 = unable to ambulate
Blood pressure
2 = systolic blood pressure +/– ≤ 20% of preanesthetic/procedural sedation level
1 = systolic blood pressure +/– ≤ 30% of preanesthetic/procedural sedation level
0 = systolic blood pressure +/– > 30% of preanesthetic/procedural sedation level
Heart rate
2 = 60–100 or if outside range, ≤ to 10% change from baseline HR
1 = outside of the range of 60–100 and the change from baseline is >10% and ≤ 20%
0 = outside of the range of 60–100 and the change from baseline is >20%
Oxygen saturation status
2 = saturation > 92% on room air, or pre preanesthetic/procedural sedation level
1 = saturation > 92% on supplemental oxygen not involving IV PCA
0 = saturation < 92% on supplemental oxygen
Pain
2 = none or mild pain with/without analgesics
1 = moderate pain controlled with analgesics
0 = persistent severe pain uncontrolled with analgesics
Postoperative nausea/vomiting
2 = none or mild nausea with no active vomiting
1 = moderate nausea or transient vomiting
0 = persistent severe nausea or vomiting
Bleeding
2 = minimal or no dressing changes
1 = moderate—Up to two dressing changes required
0 = severe—≥ three dressing changes

Acceptable discharge score is considered achieved at ≥14 provided that no individual score is 0. Any score <14 would result in either re-evaluation after achieving improvement in the suboptimal parameter

commonly used modification of the PADSS system is shown in Table 14.5 [9]. At our institution, we use a phase 2 discharge scoring tool for procedures performed in ambulatory areas as described in Table 14.5.

Fast-tracking criteria allow patients to bypass phase 1 care. Patients must meet discharge criteria to illustrate completion of phase 1 recovery before transfer from the procedure room to the ambulatory area. An example is White et al.'s fast-tracking criteria, whereby patients must meet a score of minimum of 12 out of 14, with no score <1 in any parameter [10]. Our institution has a similar fast-tracking scoring criterion available for review in Table 14.6.

Table 14.6 Cleveland Clinic fast-track criteria

Fast-tracking (PACU bypass) eligibility criteria
A score ≥18 is required for PACU discharge/bypass with no category with a score of 0.
1 Physical activity (excludes extremity with peripheral nerve block)
A. For cases done using monitored anesthesia care or general anesthesia
2 = able to move all extremities (or return to baseline)
1 = some weakness in movement of extremities
0 = no movement
B. For cases done using central neuraxial anesthesia
2 = gross motor movement of all 4 extremities (or return to baseline motor function) with return of sensory level to L5
1 = 2 segment regression of central neuraxial anesthesia and return of sensory level to L1
0 = < 2 segment regression of central neuraxial anesthesia or sensory level above L1
2 Level of consciousness
2 = fully awake
1 = arousable with verbal or tactile stimulation
0 = unresponsive
3 Blood pressure
2 = systolic blood pressure +/– 20% of preanesthetic level
1 = systolic blood pressure +/– 21–30% of preanesthetic level
0 = systolic blood pressure +/– > 30% of preanesthetic level
4 Heart rate
2 = 60 to 100 or if outside this range, ≤ 10% change from baseline HR
1 = HR outside the range of 60 to 100 and the change from baseline is >10% and ≤ 20%
0 = HR outside the range of 60 to 100 and the change from baseline is >20%
5 oxygen saturation
2 = SpO_2 ≥ 92% on room air or on supplemental oxygen with IVPCA
1 = SpO_2 ≥ 92% on supplemental oxygen not involving IVPCA
0 = SpO_2 < 92% on supplemental oxygen
6 respiration
2 = able to breathe or cough freely
1 = shallow breathing or coughing, maintains airway without support
0 = Apnea, dyspnea, tachypnea (RR >24), or bradypnea (RR <8), or requires airway support
7 pain
2 = no or mild pain with or without analgesics
1 = moderate pain controlled with analgesics
0 = persistent severe pain uncontrolled with analgesics
8 Postoperative nausea/vomiting
2 = no or mild nausea with no active vomiting
1 = moderate nausea or transient vomiting
0 = persistent severe nausea or vomiting
9 Temperature (tympanic)
2 = 36.0 ° C to 38.0 °C
1 = 35.5 °C—35.9 °C or 38.1 °C to 38.3 °C
0 = < 35.5 ° C or > 38.3 °C
10 Bleeding
2 = dry dressing, no drainage or oozing
1 = minimal oozing or drainage
0 = active bleeding, blood-soaked surgical dressing, surgical drains filling with blood (>25 ml

14.4 Discharge and Ride Status

As stated, a mandatory minimum stay should not be required prior to discharge.

Discharge with a "responsible individual" to accompany a patient home remains prudent practice. The most important description of a responsible individual is one who can report any postprocedure/postanesthesia complications. The ability to drive is not a prerequisite; however, it may be necessary to ascertain whether the mode of transportation is safe for the patient. The patient cannot be the driver; however, taking a taxi while accompanied by a responsible individual may be an acceptable option. The caregiver should understand that the patient should not be left alone for the first 12–24 h depending on the procedure and type of sedation. If there is any question as to whether the patient has a safe ride home or adequate home support, admission to the hospital should be considered [2].

14.5 Complications

Complications in PACU can be procedure related or anesthesia related. Hines et al. demonstrated a PACU complication rate of 23.7%, with the most frequent events being postoperative nausea and vomiting (PONV) [11]. Many of the postbronchoscopic complications seen in PACU are like those seen in a regular surgical PACU, albeit at a much lower incidence, and can include.

Cardiovascular

- Hypotension
- Myocardial infarction/ischemia
- Hypertension
- Hypovolemia
- Arrhythmias
- Pulmonary embolism
- CHF
- Bleeding

Respiratory

- Pneumothorax
- Upper airway obstruction
- Hypoventilation
- Hypoxemia
- Hypercapnia
- Aspiration
- Asthma/COPD exacerbation
- Pulmonary edema
- Atelectasis
- Laryngospasm
- Stridor

Neurological
- Residual muscle relaxant
- Anxiety
- Emergence delirium
- Delayed awakening
- CVA
- Seizure

Others
- Sore throat
- Pain
- PONV
- Shivering
- Hypo/hyperthermia
- Corneal abrasion
- Postop urinary retention
- Anaphylaxis

Complications More Often Seen in Bronchoscopic Procedures Include
- Excessive coughing
- Respiratory insufficiency
- Atelectasis
- Bronchospasm
- Pneumothorax
- Airway bleeding

14.6 Postoperative Nausea and Vomiting (PONV)

PONV is one of the most common postoperative problems leading to delays in discharge and increased hospital admissions. As bronchoscopic cases are mostly ambulatory cases, avoidance of PONV, which can delay discharge, may lead to hospital admission, and most definitely distress patients should be avoided. Most bronchoscopic procedures are performed with total intravenous anesthesia (TIVA), commonly a propofol infusion. Narcotics are rarely required for these procedures as pain is not a significant component. Thus, there is a decreased overall likelihood of suffering from PONV postbronschopic procedures. In addition to PONV risk mitigation strategies (avoiding inhalational anesthetic, nitrous oxide, avoiding postop narcotics) and the preventive efforts like employing a TIVA technique, it is still prudent to administer prophylactic antiemetics in all patients, especially those at higher risk [12]. Should PONV occur in the PACU, an antiemetic from a different class than that used for prophylaxis should be administered. Some options include

- 5HT-3 antagonists (serotonergic)—granisetron, ondansetron, dolasetron, tropisetron
- D2 (dopaminergic) antagonists—prochlorperazine (phenothiazine class); metoclopramide (benzamide class); droperidol, haloperidol (butyrophenone class), and amisulpride
- H1 (histamine) antagonists—diphenhydramine, promethazine
- Neurokinin NK-1 antagonist—aprepitant

14.7 Excessive Coughing

Bronchoscopy often leads to excessive coughing in the recovery room due to irritation of the airways from the bronchoscope or airway device or due to distal irritation because of needle puncture sites and bleeding. This can be troublesome and distressing for the patient. A preventive strategy of administering 100 mcg of fentanyl with induction may be utilized. It is usually self-resolving; however, if it becomes prolonged despite or in the absence of prior intraoperative fentanyl administration, it can be treated with small intravenous doses of fentanyl, IV lidocaine (0.5–1 mg/kg), or nebulized lidocaine. Of note, if a patient received lidocaine on the airway in nebulized form or by direct application, they should be cautious as they resume PO intake for a theoretical risk of aspiration.

14.8 Respiratory Complications

By nature of the fact that the procedure is performed on the airway, respiratory complications may be more frequent after bronchsocopic procedures and can range from bronchospasm, airway obstruction, hypoventilation, atelectasis, pneumothorax, or respiratory failure. When respiratory failure occurs in the PACU, one must always entertain the possibility of residual neuromuscular blockade. Patients with Eaton–Lambert syndrome, which can be associated with lung cancer, have an increased sensitivity to muscle relaxants. Pneumothorax occurs most often with sampling of the station 2 lymph nodes or peripheral lung lesions. It can present during the procedure or in the recovery room. It may present with hypoxemia, respiratory failure, chest pain, or cardiovascular collapse in case of tension pneumothorax. Pneumothorax can be detected by ultrasound, chest X-ray, or fluoroscopy. Lung atelectasis may occur from bleeding into the alveoli or excessive suctioning of the airway, leading to alveolar collapse due to negative pressure. Bleeding may occur due to multiple needle puncture sites during biopsy. Laryngospasm most often occurs during emergence but may also occur in PACU. It is often due to irritation of the vocal cords because of movement of the bronchoscope. In our experience, laryngospasm most often happens during emergence when the patient is in a light plane of anesthesia and muscle strength has returned typically in conjunction with the use of supraglottic airways for procedures such as EBUS. Bronchospasm can also occur post procedure, often because of irritation of the airways from the bronchoscope.

The PACU providers should be prompt in recognizing impending respiratory compromise and alert the anesthesiologist/pulmonologist in a timely manner.

A small percentage of patients undergoing bronchoscopic procedures who have limited respiratory reserve may require a brief period of assistance with some form of a noninvasive positive pressure ventilation, for example, BiPAP mask, to help with respiratory recovery in the immediate postprocedure period and avoid reintubation, and/or ICU admission.

It is also our experience that patients undergoing bronchoscopic procedures often have excessive secretions due to irritation of the airways and require thorough suctioning prior to extubation. These excess secretions may also contribute to laryngospasm. An antisialogogue such as glycopyrrolate may be helpful in these situations.

14.9 Cardiovascular Complications

As with postsurgical patients, postbronchoscopic cardiovascular complications can include hypertension, hypotension, arrhythmias, myocardial ischemia, heart failure, to name a few, and should be treated accordingly. The patient population presenting for bronchoscopic procedures are often older and may have preexisting cardiovascular conditions. Due to the nature of bronchoscopic procedures, fluid administration during the procedure need not be excessive, thus postprocedure fluid overload is rare; however, one must be vigilant to its occurrence in those with limited cardiac reserve.

Chest pain postbronchoscopic procedure may present a diagnostic conundrum as it is not unusual for patients to complain of chest pain due to the procedure itself. If there is a high clinical suspicion of the pain being related to a cardiac origin, diagnosis and treatment of a cardiac condition should not be delayed.

14.10 Neuropsychiatric Complications

Neuropsychiatric complications post anesthesia can include delayed emergence, emergence delirium, and intraoperative awareness.

A 2015 study found that the overall incidence of emergence delirium post anesthesia to be 4.3%, but, in patients over age 70, the incidence was 10.5% [13].

Risk factors for emergence delirium include

- Use of volatile anesthetics
- Postprocedural pain
- Specific surgical procedures, such as intra-abdominal and breast surgery in adults
- Longer duration of surgery
- Male gender
- Extremes of age
- Preexisting delirium/dementia

Again, a few of these risk factors apply to bronchsocopic procedures; however, that does not preclude the occasional postprocedure delirium from occurring.

14.11 Postoperative Urinary Retention (POUR)

Rarely is postoperative urinary retention a complication or leads to discharge delay in the bronchoscopic suite as there should be no requirement for voiding postbronchoscopic procedure prior to discharge after a bronchoscopy. However, for the sake of completeness, risk factors for POUR include male sex, advanced age, history of preexisting urinary retention, neurological disease, excessive fluid administration, prolonged anesthesia, and medications such as opioids, anticholinergics, betablockers, and sympathomimetic [14].

14.12 Conclusion

Bronchoscopic procedures may be performed under moderate or deep sedation or under general anesthesia. Although bronchoscopic procedures are quite different from surgical procedures, the same principles for monitoring and care for in recovery still apply. Regardless of the type of anesthesia used, patients must be monitored and cared for in a PACU that can provide both phase 1 and 2 recovery. Adherence to ASA guidelines for PACU patient assessment and monitoring is imperative. Often these patients transition quickly from phase 1 to phase 2 care frequently before they even leave the procedure room. This can be in part due to the nature of the bronchoscopic procedure and the rapid-acting anesthetics that are often used. A robust and safe discharge scoring tool should be used to ensure the patient is safe and "street fit" before discharging home.

As well as general postanesthetic care issues, the PACU providers should have a high index of suspicion for postprocedure complications that are more likely to occur postbronchoscopic procedures such as pneumothorax, airway bleeding, and respiratory compromise and be quick to alert the primary provider should any of these occur.

Patient should be given clear instructions on follow-up from their procedure as well as instructions on potential complications that they should be aware of post procedure.

References

1. https://www.aspan.org/Portals/88/Clinical%20Practice/FAQs/What%20are%20the%20differences%20between%20Phase%20I%20Phase%20II%20and%20Extended%20Care.pdf?ver=2020-08-14-125051-037
2. Apfelbaum JL, Silverstein JH, Chung FF, Connis RT, Fillmore RB, Hunt SE, Nickinovich DG, Schreiner MS, Silverstein JH, Apfelbaum JL, Barlow JC, Chung FF, Connis RT, Fillmore RB, Hunt SE, Joas TA, Nickinovich DG, Schreiner MS, American Society of Anesthesiologists Task Force on Postanesthetic Care. Practice guidelines for postanesthetic care: an updated report by the American Society of Anesthesiologists Task Force on Postanesthetic Care. Anesthesiology. 2013;118(2):291–307.
3. Peri anesthesia nursing standards practice recommendations and interpretive statement. 2019–2020. Cherry Hill: ASPAN; 2018.

4. Abdelmalak BB, Adhami T, Simmons W, Menendez P, Haggerty E, Troianos C. A blue print for success: implementation of the Center for Medicare and Medicaid Services (CMS) mandated anesthesiology oversight for procedural sedation in a large health system. Anesth Analg. 2022;135(1):198–208.
5. American Society of Peri Anesthesia Nurses. Perianesthesia Nursing Standards, Practive Recommendations, and Interpretive Statements. Patient Classification/ Staffing recommendations. Updated Oct 2021. https://www.aspan.org/Portals/88/Clinical%20Practice/Practice%20Recommendations/PR_Patient_Classification_Staffing_Recommendations.pdf?ver=zspJsb1KSSaT1XdIorR3Mw%3d%3d.
6. Aldrete JA, Kroulik D. A postanesthetic recovery score. Anesth Analg. 1970;49:924.
7. Aldrete JA. The post-anesthesia recovery score revisited. J Clin Anesth. 1995;7:89.
8. Chung F, Chan VW, Ong D. A post-anesthetic discharge scoring system for home readiness after ambulatory surgery. J Clin Anesth. 1995;7(6):500–6.
9. Chung F. Are discharge criteria changing? J Clin Anesth. 1993;5(6 Suppl 1):64S–8S. https://doi.org/10.1016/0952-8180(93)90011-3.
10. White PF, Song D. New criteria for fast-tracking after outpatient anesthesia: a comparison with the modified Aldrete's scoring system. Anesth Analg. 1999;88:1069.
11. Hines R, Barash PG, Watrous G, O'Connor T. Complications occurring in the postanesthesia care unit: a survey. Anesth Analg. 1992;74(4):503–9.
12. Gan TJ, Belani KG, Bergese S, Chung F, Diemunsch P, Habib AS, Jin Z, Kovac AL, Meyer TA, Urman RD, Apfel CC, Ayad S, Beagley L, Candiotti K, Englesakis M, Hedrick TL, Kranke P, Lee S, Lipman D, Minkowitz HS, Morton J, Philip BK. Fourth consensus guidelines for the management of postoperative nausea and vomiting. Anesth Analg. 2020;131(2):411–48. Erratum in: Anesth Analg. 2020;131(5):e241.
13. Wei B, Feng Y, Chen W, Ren D, Xiao D, Chen B. Risk factors for emergence agitation in adults after general anesthesia: a systematic review and meta-analysis. Acta Anaesthesiol Scand. 2021;65(6):719–29.
14. Baldini G, Bagry H, Aprikian A, Carli F. Postoperative urinary retention: anesthetic and perioperative considerations. Anesthesiology. 2009;110(5):1139–57.

Shaping the Future of Anesthesia in Interventional Pulmonology

15

Georgie Eapen

It is quite safe to state that the future of interventional pulmonology (IP) is inextricably linked with the future of interventional pulmonary anesthesia (IPA). Interventional pulmonology (IP) is an evolving subspecialty within pulmonary medicine, which is procedurally focused and simulates a hybrid practice of pulmonary medicine and thoracic surgery. While no surgeon would seriously contemplate performing thoracic surgery without the assistance of trained thoracic anesthesiologists, interventional pulmonologists often lack such focused support. The increasingly complex minimally invasive procedures being performed by interventional pulmonologists are made possible only by close collaboration with the anesthesiologist and require a similar evolution in this subspecialty of anesthesiology. Shaping the future of IP will be impossible without concurrent advancements in anesthesia techniques, management strategies, patient safety protocols, technological innovations, and extensive interdisciplinary collaboration.

Historically, IP procedures primarily involved flexible bronchoscopy, which could be carried out under moderate sedation, often administered by the bronchoscopist. Recent decades have seen a significant expansion of more sophisticated techniques such as endobronchial ultrasound (EBUS), rigid bronchoscopy, robotic-assisted bronchoscopy, and medical thoracoscopy becoming widespread. Each advance presents unique challenges and requires an evolution in anesthesia management to optimize patient outcomes and procedural efficiency. The modification of anesthesia techniques reflects growing procedural length and complexity, progressing from moderate sedation for simpler interventions to general anesthesia for advanced procedures like rigid bronchoscopy and robotic-assisted interventions [5].

The significant uptake in IP procedure has been underpinned by more widespread adoption of general anesthesia, which is critical in providing patient comfort,

G. Eapen (✉)
Department of Pulmonary Medicine, The University of Texas MD Anderson Cancer Center, Houston, TX, USA
e-mail: geapen@mdanderson.org

M. Sarkiss (ed.), *Anesthesia for Interventional Pulmonary Procedures*,
https://doi.org/10.1007/978-3-032-12007-6_15

airway protection, optimal procedural conditions, and ensuring effective ventilation strategies. Advanced collaborative airway management techniques tailored to specific IP procedures—such as airway stenting or massive hemoptysis management—highlight the increasing expertise required from anesthesiologists in this field. Enhanced ventilation modes, such as jet ventilation and tailored mechanical ventilation strategies, continue to evolve, emphasizing patient safety and procedural success [3].

Regional anesthesia is also playing an increasing role by providing alternatives for chest wall interventions and pleural procedures. Understanding thoracic anatomy and developing minimally invasive regional blocks, such as paravertebral and intercostal nerve blocks, allows for targeted pain management that decrease systemic anesthetic requirements, resulting in minimally invasive procedures, shorter recovery periods, decreased postoperative complications, and enhanced patient comfort [7].

Preoperative patient assessment and optimization are also an integral component of IP anesthesia. Comprehensive evaluations include detailed cardiopulmonary examinations, airway assessments, functional testing, and risk stratifications. High-risk conditions such as chronic obstructive pulmonary disease (COPD), pulmonary hypertension, anemia, electrolyte derangements, and malnutrition require early identification and targeted management strategies to optimize patient outcomes. Programs for smoking cessation, pulmonary rehabilitation, and vaccinations may further enhance patient readiness, significantly improving procedural success and recovery profiles [6].

Technological innovations, notably robotic bronchoscopy, highlight another transformative aspect of IP anesthesia. Robotic-assisted procedures require specialized anesthetic strategies to accommodate technical complexities and prolonged procedural durations. Ventilatory strategies profoundly affect CT to body divergence, impacting diagnostic accuracy. Anesthesiologists must therefore expertly manage the unique airway and ventilation challenges posed by robotic systems, partnering closely with the interventional pulmonologist to achieve technical success and field innovative clinical care. These collaborative deployments of the robotic technologies promise greater precision, reduced complications, and expanded therapeutic capabilities within IP [1].

Patient safety continues to be paramount, guiding enhancements in preoperative assessment, intraoperative management, and postoperative recovery and monitoring protocols. Evidence-based anesthetic and opioid use and judicious neuromuscular blockade are critical for avoiding perioperative complications. Vigilant postoperative care includes structured recovery room criteria, standardized monitoring for respiratory and cardiovascular complications, and proactive management of common postoperative issues such as nausea, excessive coughing, and urinary retention. Robust recovery and discharge protocols ensure safe, efficient patient transitions from anesthesia to discharge, minimizing complications and improving overall patient satisfaction [2].

The integration of personalized medicine and artificial intelligence (AI) likely represents the future of anesthesia in IP. AI-driven predictive analytics may facilitate precise risk stratification, tailored anesthetic techniques, and proactive complication management. Such personalized approaches could enhance patient outcomes, reduce procedural risks, and streamline healthcare delivery, marking a significant shift toward precision medicine in IP anesthesia [4]. Research efforts should be continuously directed toward the development and incorporation of evidence-based clinical practice.

Educational initiatives and interdisciplinary collaboration are also essential for continued innovation in IP anesthesia. Specialized training programs designed explicitly for anesthesiologists in IP, incorporating simulation-based learning and interdisciplinary case discussions, may aid in developing expertise and fostering innovation. Collaborative efforts among interventional pulmonologists, anesthesiologists, nurses, and bronchoscopy technicians are vital to foster a robust environment for innovation, education, and excellence in patient care [8].

In conclusion, shaping the future of anesthesia in interventional pulmonology involves embracing advanced and evolving procedural techniques, continuously refining anesthetic strategies while prioritizing patient safety through innovative technologies, and fostering educational collaborations. These efforts are all ultimately predicated on the recognition that much like IP is a distinct subspecialty of pulmonary medicine, IP anesthesia is a distinct subspecialty of anesthesia. Taken together, these efforts promise to significantly enhance patient care, procedural outcomes, and the overall scope and effectiveness of interventional pulmonology.

References

1. Agrawal A, Hogarth DK, Murgu S. Robotic bronchoscopy for pulmonary lesions: a review. J Thorac Dis. 2020;12(6):3279–86.
2. Apfelbaum JL, Silverstein JH, Chung FF, Connis RT, Fillmore RB. Practice guidelines for postanesthetic care. Anesthesiology. 2013;118(2):291–307.
3. Colt HG, Dumon JF. Airway stents: present and future. Clin Chest Med. 1992;13(2):231–43.
4. Connor CW. Artificial intelligence and machine learning in anesthesiology. Anesthesiology. 2019;131(6):1346–59.
5. Ernst A, Silvestri GA. Interventional pulmonology procedures: guidelines from the American College of Chest Physicians. Chest. 2009;135(4):1118–26.
6. Kaplan JA, Slinger PD, Fraser WD. Thoracic anesthesia. 3rd ed. Elsevier Health Sciences; 2008.
7. Karmakar MK. Thoracic paravertebral block. Anesthesiology. 2001;95(3):771–80.
8. Wahidi MM, Lamb C, Murgu S, et al. American Association for Bronchology and Interventional Pulmonology statement on training in interventional pulmonology. Respirology. 2020;25(6):566–73.

Index

M. Sarkiss (ed.), *Anesthesia for Interventional Pulmonary Procedures*, https://doi.org/10.1007/978-3-032-12007-6

MIX
Papier aus verantwortungsvollen Quellen
Paper from responsible sources
FSC® C105338

If you have any concerns about our products,
you can contact us on
ProductSafety@springernature.com

In case Publisher is established outside the EU,
the EU authorized representative is:
Springer Nature Customer Service Center GmbH
Europaplatz 3, 69115 Heidelberg, Germany

Printed by Libri Plureos GmbH
in Hamburg, Germany